GOOD
MORNINGS

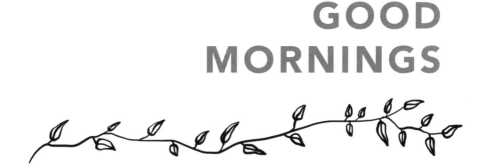

GOOD MORNINGS

MORNING RITUALS FOR WELLNESS, PEACE AND PURPOSE

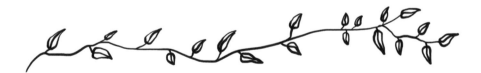

LINNEA DUNNE

An Hachette UK Company
www.hachette.co.uk

First published in Great Britain in 2019 by Gaia,
an imprint of Octopus Publishing Group Ltd
Carmelite House
50 Victoria Embankment
London EC4Y 0DZ
www.octopusbooks.co.uk
www.octopusbooksusa.com

This edition published in 2024

Distributed in the US by Hachette Book Group
1290 Avenue of the Americas
4th and 5th Floors, New York, NY 10104

Distributed in Canada by Canadian Manda Group
664 Annette St., Toronto, Ontario, Canada M6S 2C8

ISBN 978-1-85675-530-6

Printed and bound in China.

10 9 8 7 6 5 4 3 2 1

Commissioning Editor: Leanne Bryan
Senior Editor: Pollyanna Poulter
Copy Editor: Alison Wormleighton
Art Director: Juliette Norsworthy
Designer: Megan van Staden
Illustrator: Gabi Froden
Production Controller: Emily Noto

CONTENTS

"The first hour of the morning
is the rudder of the day."
— HENRY WARD BEECHER

INTRODUCTION

The magic of the morning

WAKING UP TO MAGIC

If you've ever spent a night in a tent, you'll know what it's like to wake to birdsong: that initially hesitant lilt, slowly growing into a crescendo of confident trills, so perfectly complementing the early morning mist. There is something utterly magical about such things we can't control. We know the birdsong will come, we just can't quite predict exactly when - so we wait, we pause, perfectly still. And we listen.

I have always been tuned into the sound of birds, perhaps a legacy of my school biology lessons when a stout, mustachioed teacher from way up in the north of Sweden would play cassette tapes of different bird sounds on repeat and then quiz us on them. Or, perhaps more likely, it might be due to the deeply sincere appreciation of the arrival of spring among a nation of people that grew up surrounded by thick, persistent darkness for months on end. We learned to appreciate birdsong when spring brought it to us. Perhaps, in some way, it is all linked to the Swedish tradition of *gökotta*.

While few Swedes practise *gökotta* today, the tradition lives on, among other things as part of a *"gökotta* service" in local churches on Ascension Day, followed by a stroll through the woods. Moreover, as more and more Swedes wish to reconnect with nature and cherish offline moments in an increasingly busy world, nature groups and bird-watching societies have seen a revived interest in *gökotta* experiences. Perhaps the old tradition has a very relevant thing or two to teach us.

EXPERIENCING GÖKOTTA
Picture early morning mist in Sweden at around the turn of the 20th century. Imagine the villagers in the leafy localities of the hilly county of Dalarna gathering in the woods on Ascension Day (40 days after Easter) and during the build-up to midsummer. Together, the villagers would listen to the first of the morning's birdsong, in particular the cuckoo – *gök* in Swedish (*otta* means "early morning", so *gökotta* means "early morning cuckoo"). Some would bring a Thermos of coffee or stay for a picnic in the park.

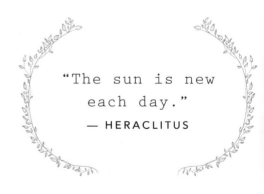

"The sun is new each day."
— HERACLITUS

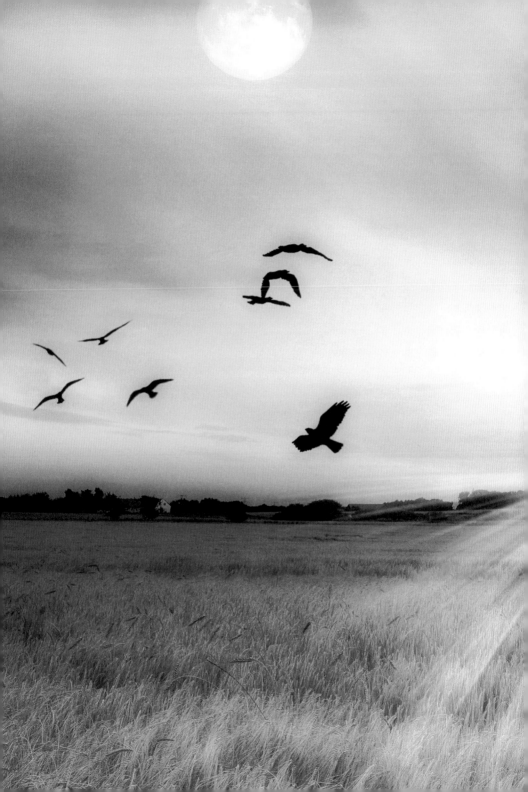

"Early to bed and early to
rise makes a man healthy,
wealthy and wise."
— BENJAMIN FRANKLIN

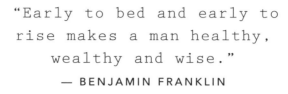

POSITIVE PROOF FROM THE TOP OF THE MOST SUCCESSFUL COMPANIES

In business and personal development circles, the morning ritual is quickly becoming a must. It's not for nothing that successful business people such as Robert Iger, CEO of Disney, and Tim Cook, CEO of Apple, rise at 4.30am and 5am respectively. Indeed, the ancient Greek philosopher Aristotle once said, "It is well to be up before daybreak, for such habits contribute to health, wealth and wisdom." Although we focus less on material riches in this book, the sentiment certainly resonates.

RITUALS OF THE BIG SHOTS

In fact, the list goes on. Barack and Michelle Obama rise early for daily exercise, and Bill Gates, co-founder of Microsoft, starts the day with exercise for both body and mind. Arianna Huffington, co-founder of the *Huffington Post*, has spoken about a morning ritual of deep breathing, gratitude and intention setting – one that, crucially, is entirely cell phone-free. Howard Schultz, former CEO of Starbucks, gets up at dawn every morning to walk his dog, then has a special grind of coffee with his wife. The late Steve Jobs is said to have started each day by looking at himself in the mirror and asking, "If today were the last day of my life, would I be happy with what I'm about to do today?".

THE SCIENCE OF RISING EARLY

But don't just take the big-shot CEOs' word for it. Science and biology are here to back up the benefits of rising early.

Our circadian rhythm (also known as our internal body clock) is regulated by daylight, which is why going to bed early and rising early has been shown to contribute to better sleep. What we eat and drink – or refrain from eating and drinking – in the morning tells our body and metabolism how to behave for the rest of the day (for more on this, see chapter 5).

Morning exercise can increase concentration and motivation throughout the day (see page 67), not to mention the fact that a dip in the cold sea or a run in the fresh air certainly wakes the body up and makes you feel alive. And that's in addition to the many health benefits of spending time in nature (see chapter 7).

Practising optimism and gratitude, meanwhile, has a similar effect on the brain to taking antidepressants (see page 96). How much more proof do we need in order to end that unhealthy relationship with the snooze button?

RECLAIM THE MORNING

I once heard someone describe the morning as the seed that blossoms into what becomes your day. I think, for many of us, it's true. That feeling when you run for the bus and miss it; the guilt of starting the day by snapping at your kids; the dismay as you realize your shirt needs ironing but you don't have time - those feelings linger. But so, too, do the positive, empowering moments.

BEING PRESENT HERE AND NOW

In a world of "always on", a world expecting us to dwell on the past or worry about the future, a world of 24/7 notifications and counting likes on Instagram, choosing to be present here and now is quite the radical act. Yet, without that presence, how could you possibly deal with the unpredictability of modern life? It's that very choice, the commitment to being with ourselves, fully, if only for a short moment every morning, that helps us take notice of our inner compass and trust that we are able to deal with whatever comes our way.

THE GOLDEN PROMISE OF WHAT'S YET TO BE DETERMINED

"The early bird catches the worm," goes the old English proverb. Indeed, you could think of it as a way to be one step ahead, to have cleared the deck before the working day even begins. But, as a Swede, I prefer the Swedish metaphor *morgonstund har guld i mun*, meaning "morning time has gold in its mouth". You need to rise early to notice, but the beauty is not so much in the victory as in the discovery, in the dedication and commitment to seeing what's there: the shadows cast by those early morning rays, the silence of a house still asleep, the promise of a city that's only just waking up.

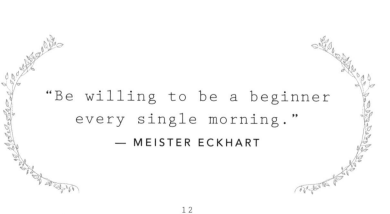

"Be willing to be a beginner every single morning."
— MEISTER ECKHART

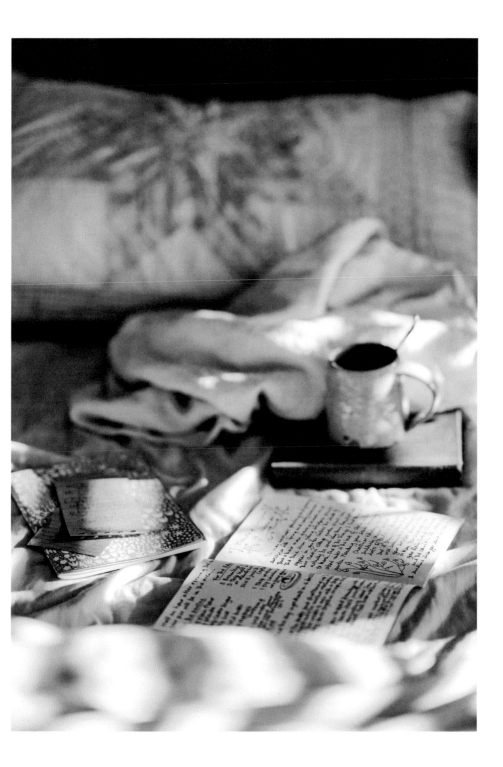

"We turn not older with years,
but newer every day."
— EMILY DICKINSON

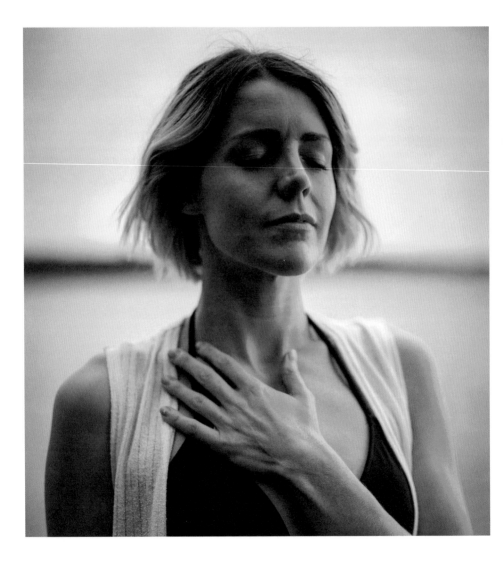

CARVING OUT TIME TO LISTEN TO YOURSELF

The idea of starting each day with birdsong may sound overly romantic, but incorporating an element of peaceful ritual into our morning routine doesn't have to be difficult. With work starting increasingly early, often on the commute, and chores leaving little space for "me time" in the evenings, more and more of us are choosing to set aside a portion of every day as an almost-sacred time - a time for checking in with ourselves and our world without interruption.

Some people see their morning ritual as a conscious choice to reclaim their individuality – not necessarily for the benefit of self-development and self-realization, but as a healthy commitment to their own wellbeing through the investment of time and awareness. How often have you heard people express surprise at their own burnout or depression? They were fine and then they were fine again and then still fine – until suddenly they were not. They had been too busy to notice the warning signs.

RITUALS FOR AVOIDING FRICTION

Small things like frantically looking for your keys might not seem significant enough to change the infrastructure of your entire morning, but keen morning ritualists have started trying to erase this so-called friction from their day. Not only do they make sure things like keys are in their designated places,

but they also adopt habits like creating a capsule wardrobe and eating the same thing every morning. By removing the need to make these everyday decisions, they leave more space for the person underneath to emerge.

THE KEY TO UNLOCKING YOUR DAY

It's not easy to check in with yourself and get an honest answer in between replying to messages and making phone calls. But the freshness of the morning provides that opportunity: a chance to be fully present as you open the door, to really feel how you are carrying yourself as you step into your day.

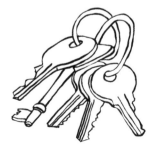

HOW TO BECOME A MORNING PERSON

I believe in self-kindness, and I believe in doing what works - and I don't think rising at dawn necessarily needs to be the goal you're striving for if getting out of bed early in the morning makes you miserable. That said, if you are going to add a morning ritual to your everyday life, you will at least need to find a way to get up earlier.

Night owls *can* become early birds. It has happened before, and successfully, too. The reality is that, although changing the rhythm of the day can be tough at the start, very few people stop rising early once they've started. Do you want in on their secret? Motivation is key, but a little strategy also goes a long way. Here are a few tried-and-tested tips to get you started.

ASK YOURSELF "WHY?"
Ignoring what other people tell you, think about why you want to change. Picture that time set aside for yourself – imagine the peace and quiet or that feeling you'll have after some morning yoga. Try to paint a vivid picture for yourself.

IDENTIFY AND REMEDY OBSTACLES
Consider the reasons why the idea of rising early makes your head hurt. That feeling of getting out from underneath the duvet and putting your feet on the cold floor can be relieved by bringing your slippers to the bedside at night or setting the heating to come on a little earlier. The sheer exhaustion can be counteracted by making sure that you

sleep during the most important hours, starting at around 11pm when melatonin (a hormone that regulates sleep) peaks. It will take willpower, of course – you might need to remind yourself of those good reasons for doing it that you identified when you asked yourself "why?".

CHANGE YOUR ALARM
The snooze function on an alarm is a night owl's best friend and an early bird's worst enemy. Moreover, sleeping right next to the alarm has all sorts of negative effects, from disturbed sleep to (in the case of sleeping next to your cell phone) potential links to some forms of cancer. Some people advocate a cold-turkey approach, leaving their alarm in a different room so that they have to get out of bed to turn it off. Whether you do that or not, make sure the alarm sounds pleasant rather than loud and strident – there's a lot to be said for waking up to your favourite tune.

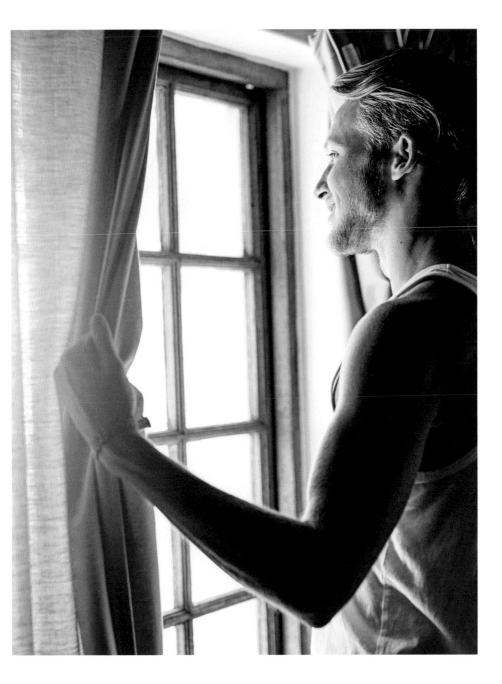

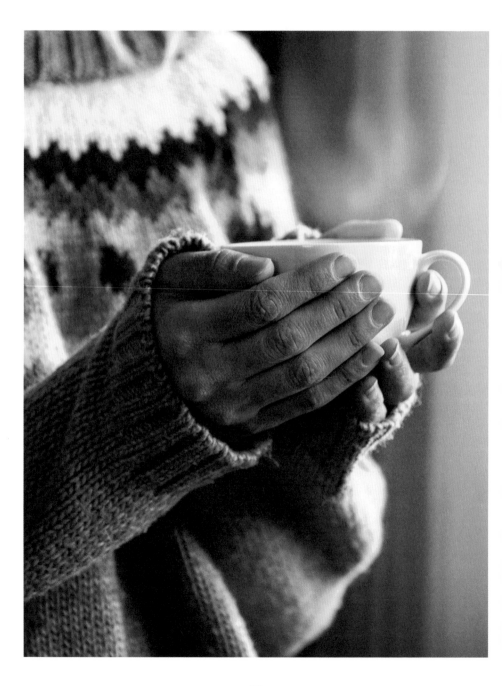

MOTIVATION FROM WITHIN

When I was 11, I had a headache every Thursday morning. It just so happened that Thursday was violin lesson day and I knew that, if I was unwell enough to stay home from school, I wouldn't be made to go to my violin lesson. By the time I turned 13, I'd stopped playing the violin altogether.

The lesson in this? Motivation can't be handed down. This book provides inspiration, ideas and support, but the motivation must come from within. If you picked up this book, you are probably hoping for some aspect of your life to change and thinking that starting each day a little differently might be a good step. Keep that in mind as you read through – remember why you picked it up in the first place.

The more I read and speak to people, the more convinced I am that a little awareness goes a long way, and that having time for reflection can make us happier and more grounded. But does that mean that everyone should get up at dawn? Probably not.

THE IMPORTANCE OF SELF-CARE

There will be things in this book that don't speak to you and that you would never do. Skip those pages if you want – not everyone was made for an early morning workout. If you design your morning ritual to please someone else, or as some notion of what self-care *should* look like, you're not going to keep it up – and it probably doesn't qualify as self-care anyway.

TREAT YOURSELF WITH SELF-KINDNESS

I once heard someone say that love is meeting in the middle. I think we could all do with meeting *ourselves* in the middle – forgiving ourselves if we can't do it all. That's what self-care is: it's not about choosing to be happy, but choosing to try. You don't have to be the best version of yourself every single day – but you can try your best, all the time. That halfway point represents self-kindness and compassion. If more of us were able to find that sweet spot, what a world we could live in.

> "Magic is believing in yourself. If you can do that, you can make anything happen."
> — JOHANN WOLFGANG VON GOETHE

"You are not a drop in the ocean.
You are the entire ocean, in a drop."

— RUMI

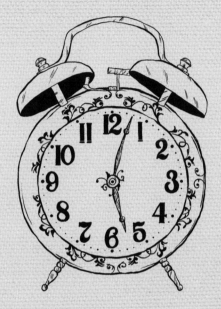

CHAPTER 1

COMMIT

What's in a ritual?

TAKING COMFORT IN RITUAL

When I was a child, it was important to me that my family's Christmas traditions were played out in exactly the same way every year. I vividly remember the upset when it was suggested that we change the day we decorate the Christmas tree. Impossible! It wouldn't have seemed like Christmas at all. You could say that I was taking comfort in the ritual. It was a fun celebration, but it had to be followed, consciously and with effort and full presence, in a predictable way.

RITUAL THE WORLD OVER

Whether we know it or not, most of us engage in a great number of rituals in our everyday lives, particularly during special occasions. Some of us get water splashed across our heads as we are welcomed into a community of faith; some share symbols of eternity to celebrate their love for each other and the intention to stay together forever. In some communities, the arrival of the menses in young women is marked by ritual, and countless different rituals are practised every year across the globe to express gratitude for the harvest.

In my native Sweden, we jump like frogs around a phallic-looking floral maypole at midsummer and, when graduating from secondary school, we wear sailor hats. When I was growing up, my family embraced the common activity known in Sweden as *fredagsmys* or "cosy Friday". Every Friday evening we would sit in front of the television, sharing a special spread of dips, vegetable sticks and potato chips plus a rare bottle of soda pop. Every birthday, we woke up to a chair decorated with the flowers of the season and a Swedish flag made of wood beside our breakfast plate.

TIMELESS PRACTICES

The word *ritual* might spark associations with everything from the sacrificing of animals to deeply religious and sometimes secretive traditions. But looking at how communities and societies have developed and expressed themselves, it becomes clear that a ritual can be much more than that – and it is just as central to life today as it was to long-gone tribes and our religious forefathers.

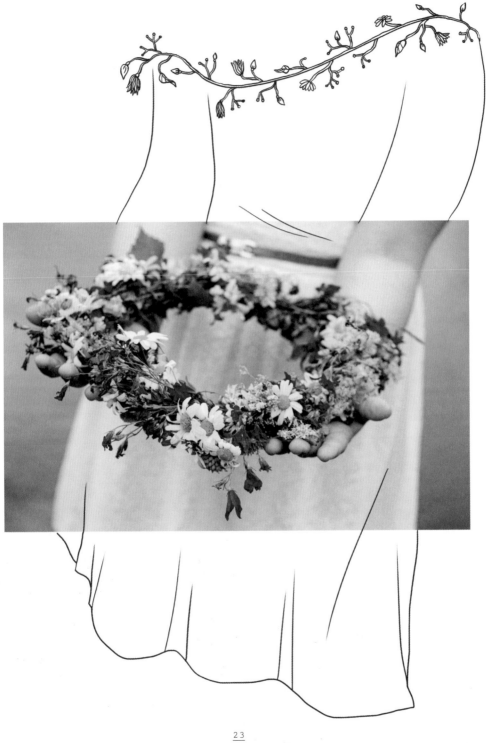

"There is a morning inside you
waiting to burst open into light."
— RUMI

RITUAL AS AGENCY

---

*When I was 15, I spent a month at a Christian summer camp.
Each morning at 7am we met in the chapel before breakfast for
a silent prayer or a song on repeat, harmonizing (and yawning -
some were in pyjamas still). There were candles everywhere,
and no talking. The hardwood floor creaked as you walked on it,
or when sitting down; there weren't enough seats for everyone,
but no one minded. Some were hugging, some closing their eyes.
I don't know if there was a divine presence - there wasn't for
me - yet it was certainly a morning ritual for the soul.*

RITUAL IN MAGICAL, SACRED SPACES

In a podcast that I listened to recently, two Swedish folk musicians spoke about magical spaces: chapels, convents, forests, remote huts and shacks. Some were places in which women historically were allowed to just be together, without getting married or having children and homes to mind – cracks in the ordinary everyday life where there was room for something sacred, for magic. The two musicians said they think that all people of all times have had this need to create their own magical spaces, just to cope with life.

RITUAL AS INTENTIONAL LIVING

I think this notion of ritual as agency is true for rituals past and present: they represent a conscious effort to make sense of life and to claim our space. It would be easy to think of rituals performed by entire communities as mechanical groupthink, but look at indigenous peoples holding on to rituals in the face of modernization; workers who keep marching and chanting as an entire global economic system denies their value; groups of people meditating silently in the middle of the unending noise of the surrounding city. This is intentional living.

RITUAL AS AN ACT OF RESISTANCE

I believe, as some scholars have argued, that ritual can be an act of resistance, a creative anti-structure, a refusal to conform and an insistence that I am the creator of me and that I, no matter what, will speak my truth.

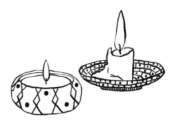

RITUAL AS WE KNOW IT

We have always used ritual to express shared values and make sense of life at critical junctures. As human beings, we seem to favour familiar, habitual activities to help us put emotions into context and create a language and platform for sharing experiences with each other.

RITUAL IN EVERYDAY LIFE
We may use ritual for any number of purposes:

- **Lending confidence** such as taking a moment in front of the mirror, or power-posing every time we are about to give a talk or presentation.

- **Bringing luck** for example, giving our child a high-five before they run onto the pitch ahead of a game, or wearing a special garment or good-luck charm to job interviews and challenging events.

- **Bonding** including sports teams gathering for a chant before every match.

- **Offering security and comfort** notably singing the same lullabies to children night after night, and developing patterns of doing things in a particuar order, such as fluffing up pillows and switching off lights.

- **Resisting** such as chanting collectively at protests.

- **Celebrating** through birthday traditions and songs, or performing a celebratory action when scoring a goal.

These actions are carriers of deep meaning. We find confidence in their predictability and familiarity. Perhaps it's easier to rest and feel supported in an experience we know and trust? I don't see why it would be much different when we are alone.

RITUAL AS A TOOL
Picture that magical space: a chapel, the woods, your yoga mat, perhaps a brand-new notebook. In the same way that we use ritual to check in with each other and create the conditions for collective growth in our societies and communities, so we can use it to check in with ourselves and adjust our inner compass with awareness. If we can employ ritual in this way – to acknowledge our emotions, learn to express ourselves and find renewed confidence – it could be just as useful now as it ever has been.

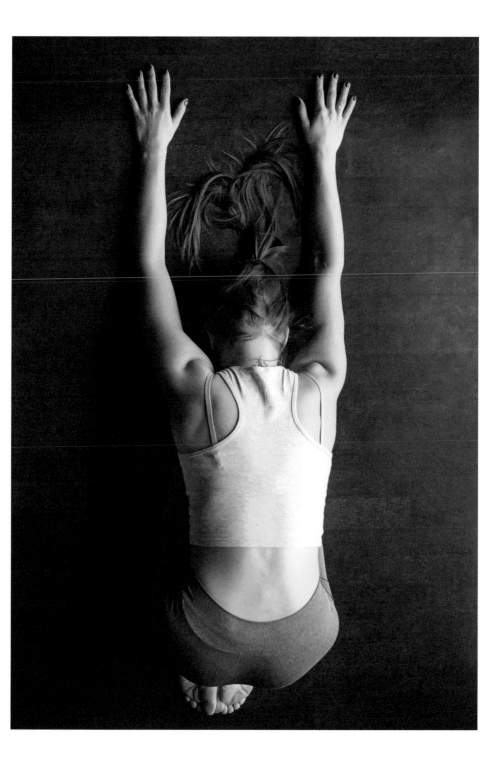

A PSYCHOLOGIST ON RITUALS AND SMALL STEPS

Aisling Leonard-Curtin is a chartered psychologist, co-author of The Power of Small *and co-director of ACT Now Purposeful Living. Here she shares her view on the importance of committing to small but regular acts of self-care for sustainable change.*

THE POWER OF SMALL STEPS

"When we set excessive expectations for ourselves, one of two things usually happens: we either find the task too overwhelming and end up procrastinating, or we start off all guns blazing and then burn out and stop. In founding ACT Now Purposeful Living we wanted to prevent people from falling into this trap, and we noticed – and this is validated by the research – that we have a better chance of making long-term, meaningful changes in our actions if we can break them into smaller chunks, which can build incrementally over time to amount to huge changes in our lives."

SUSTAINABLE PSYCHOLOGICAL CHANGE

"The majority of neuroimaging studies do not show significant changes in our neural pathways after a short period of engaging in a healthy habit. The stronger neurological changes happen when we engage in different behaviours over a sustained period of time. The Power of Small *approach gives people a better chance of long-term sustainable psychological change."*

ON COMMITTING TO DAILY BREAKOUTS

"What eventually morphed into The Power of Small *was what we called 5-minute breakouts, a tool to help people recognize their current comfort zone and then spend 5 minutes each day breaking out of it. With this approach, the comfort zone gradually and consistently expands, leading to a richer and fuller life."*

ON CONNECTING TO YOUR VALUES

"Morning rituals can be an extremely powerful way to set people up for the day ahead. When we engage in actions that bring us closer to our values and let go of actions that take us further away from them, our sense of wellness and contentment increases in the long term. Some of these daily habits can bring up some discomfort in the short term yet will ultimately be beneficial in the long term, leading to improved psychological wellbeing, a greater sense of authenticity and alignment with our inner core values and meaningful productivity, rather than busyness for the sake of busyness."

TAKE YOUR FIRST SMALL STEP

"The exercise opposite is a great place to start if you want to explore connecting (or, indeed, reconnecting) to your key values.

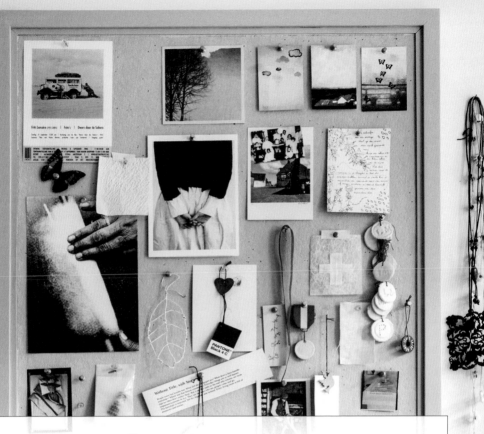

Connect to your values –
an exercise from *The Power of Small*:

1. Think of 5 values that are really important to you, such as courage and connection.

2. Find images that represent these values. Cut them out or print them off and affix them to a sheet of paper. Make the montage as visually appealing as you can.

3. Look at the sheet for 5 minutes every morning and reflect on which actions in the past 24 hours brought you closer to these values, and which took you farther away from them. Then reflect on the 24 hours ahead. Plan for any potential challenges and ways to move closer to your values despite those challenges.

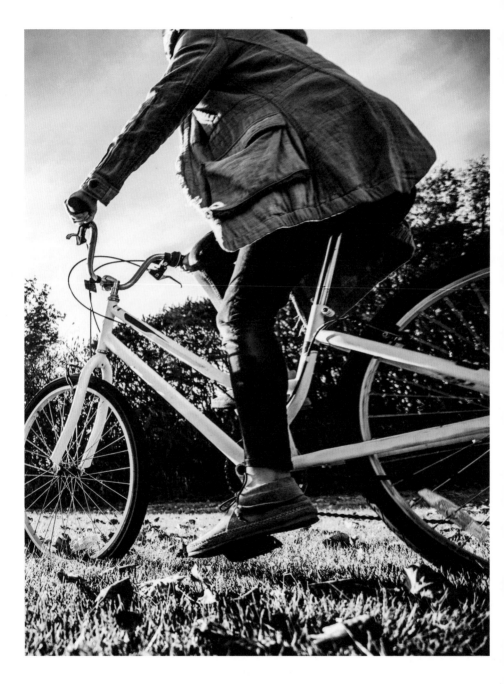

ROUTINE OR RITUAL?

*Talk to people about morning rituals and few people will
say they have one. Yet they'll be very keen to tell you
about their morning routine, perhaps including a certain
cleansing regime or having a coffee on their daily stroll
to work - and they might have quite strong feelings about
it. This, of course, begs the question, when is a routine
more than just a routine and when can you call it a ritual?*

HABITS WITH MEANING

When speaking of ritual, many people talk about an awareness and a commitment – the difference between doing something purely out of habit and doing it because it means something to you. The meaning associated with a ritual, in fact, seems to be a big factor: once you imbue an activity or sequence of actions with meaning, or when you start to feel a deep emotional attachment to it, you could probably think of it as a ritual.

Some people see the notion of ritual as either pretentious or too rooted in New Age practices. No matter how attached they are to their own early morning habits, they prefer to regard them as nothing but a mundane routine.

EMBRACING YOUR INNER HIPPIE

But we are creatures of habit; we tend to hold on to meaning wherever we can find it. Historically, ritual has been important in shaping and acknowledging identity, identifying and accepting emotions in the present moment, and carving out a vision for the future. I think that everyday rituals can remain tools for these very purposes, for us as individuals and as small parts of a greater whole. And I think you can embrace, non-judgementally, your inner hippie if you are that way inclined – or stay cynical yet take self-care very seriously all the same. The people I have met who engage in a daily ritual are all people who have promised themselves a little bit of space, a little bit of love and a fist in the air when the going gets tough. Surely that's something that we could all benefit from doing?

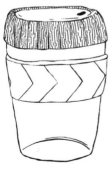

"We first make our habits,
then our habits make us."
— JOHN DRYDEN

"Where there is peace
and meditation,
there is neither
anxiety nor doubt."
— ST FRANCIS OF ASSISI

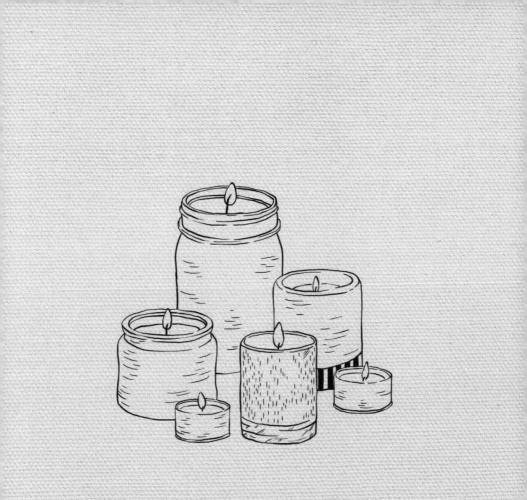

CHAPTER 2

BREATHE

Yoga and meditation rituals

THE POWER
OF THE BREATH

———————————————

*Most of us would never think of breathing as a tool. In fact,
we would probably never think of it at all. It's such a simple
thing, automatic, constant - a never-ending rhythm of life.
And yet the breath is hugely powerful, and learning to be
aware of it and to control it has been at the heart of
Eastern philosophy since ancient times.*

THE PRANAYAMA WAY

In yoga, breath control or mastery is called *pranayama*. This means in practical terms the ability to use the breath for self-awareness and to work from that awareness as needed throughout the day. The skills involved in mastering the breath are described as being threefold: identification, differentiation and integration – in other words the discipline to observe the breath, the ability to change it and the power to adapt it in a beneficial way.

BENEFITS OF MINDFUL BREATHING

There's a reason why we remind each other to take a deep breath when we feel stressed or angry or need to gather our thoughts in preparation for something we are nervous about. Mindful breathing has been proved to help with lowering anxiety and stress levels and improving mental health in general, including cognitive ability. Researchers have also found links between controlled breathing and lower blood pressure as well as improved respiratory and cardiovascular health.

WHY RELEARN HOW TO BREATHE?

As one of the most effective ways to lower stress levels, *pranayama* may help prevent everything from insomnia to panic attacks. In short, relearning how to breathe might be the best thing you've ever done. Breathing is also at the heart of meditation and yoga practices, which you can read more about in this chapter.

"There is one way of breathing that is
shameful and constricted. Then, there's
another way: a breath of love that takes
you all the way to infinity."

— RUMI

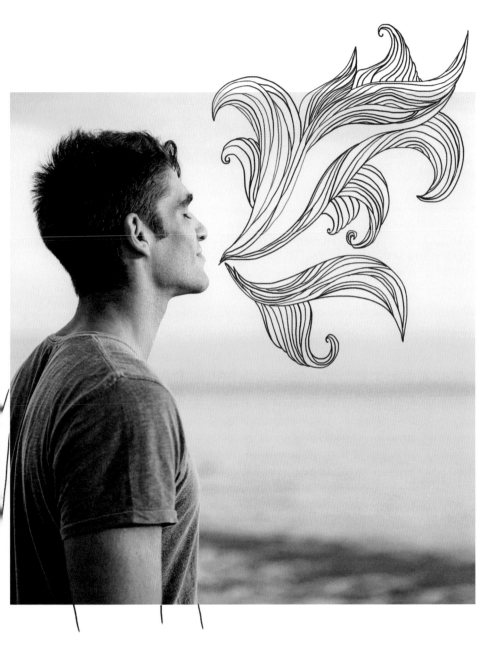

"For breath is life, and if you breathe well you will live long on earth."
— SANSKRIT PROVERB

SLOW DOWN

According to some breathing experts and coaches, our ability to breathe is underdeveloped - and becoming more so. The tendency to hold the belly in, plus poor posture, results in shallow breathing that only uses the top part of the lungs - you could say that the way we live today results in our making the least of our breathing mechanism. Not only are we missing out on all the incredible benefits of breath mastery, but by failing to breathe properly we are, in fact, doing ourselves harm.

A LITTLE BIT OF SCIENCE

You have probably heard of the body's autonomic nervous system. This governs the sympathetic and parasympathetic systems – the former is responsible for the fight-or-flight response; the latter, the rest-and-digest mode. These systems, which manage everything from heart rate to respiration and digestion, developed through evolution as a survival mechanism to enable us to respond quickly to threats (fight and flight) and then recover and restore (rest and digest). If you are an anxious person, your sympathetic nervous system is likely to be triggered a little too easily.

WHY IS THIS IMPORTANT TODAY?

Our respiratory system sends signals to the brainstem to activate the sympathetic nervous system – the more signals it sends, the faster we breathe. As the breath slows down, the parasympathetic nervous system is elicited and we start to relax. Imagine, then, that your default breathing is a little too shallow and a little too fast – and then you have to navigate the modern-day reality of cell phone notifications, pop-up windows and nonstop noise. Can you see how learning to master your breath could change everything?

Massaging the vagus nerve

The vagus nerve, also known as the tenth cranial nerve, links the brainstem to the lungs, heart and gut. Controlled breathing helps to tone this nerve, which explains why slow, deep breathing stimulates the parasympathetic nervous system for a calming effect. As such, the breath can be an important tool for effective meditation and sound mental and physical health.

GET TO KNOW YOUR BREATH

If you want to incorporate a breathing exercise into your morning ritual, one of the following methods could be a good place to start. For the first one, you need to lie down on the floor or on a yoga mat. For the other three, start by finding a comfortable seated position, possibly on a folded blanket or yoga mat to ensure that your spine is straight.

DIAPHRAGMATIC BREATHING

This technique involves contracting the diaphragm, the muscle at the base of your lungs. Associated with relaxation, it is also used by singers and wind instrument players, to get maximum oxygen into the bloodstream.
How to do it…Lying flat, place one hand on your belly below the ribcage. As you breathe, notice your belly rising and falling and try to slow down your breath to a steady but relaxed pace. Your shoulders and ribcage should remain almost still, with most of the movement taking place where you can feel it with your hand: in the diaphragm.
When and for how long…Practise for a few minutes every morning.

4-7-8 BREATHING

This breathing technique will help you to relax and clear your mind. It is also said to assist insomniacs with sleep.
How to do it…With the tip of your tongue behind your upper front teeth, just on the ridge of your gums, slowly inhale through your nose for a count of 4. Hold your breath for a count of 7, and then open your mouth slightly without moving your tongue and exhale for a count of 8. Repeat four times.
When and for how long…Whenever you like, for as long as you need to feel calm.

NADI SHODHANA BREATHING

Also known as Alternate Nostril Breathing, for reasons that will become obvious.
How to do it…Close your eyes and take a full, deep breath in, followed by a gentle breath out. Continue until your breath feels full and relaxed. Position your right hand in the gesture known as Vishnu Mudra by folding the index and middle fingers so that the tips touch the palm at the base of the thumb. Alternatively, rest your index and middle finger gently on your forehead (as shown opposite). Plug your right nostril using your right thumb and exhale gently but fully through your left nostril. With the right nostril still plugged, inhale through your left nostril. Feel your breath travel up the left side of your spine. Plug your left nostril with the ring finger and pinky finger of your right hand and release the right nostril. Exhale through the right nostril, pause and then inhale through your right nostril. This time, feel your breath travel up the right side of your spine. Plug the right

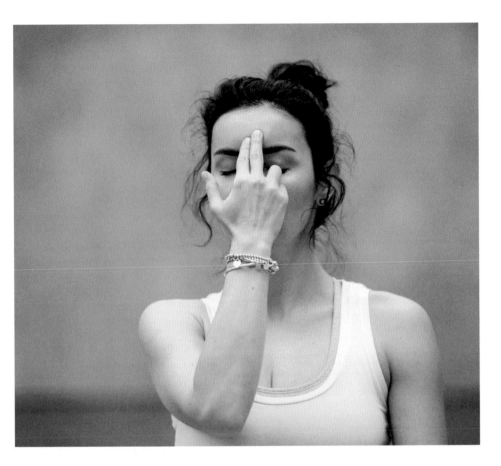

nostril again with the thumb and exhale on the left side, completing one cycle. Steadily repeat the cycle of inhale left, exhale right, inhale right and exhale left five to ten times. **When and for how long…**Best practised on an empty stomach in the early morning. This should take no more than 10 minutes.

KAPALABHATI BREATHING

Also called Skull-polishing Breath, this is one of the six cleansing practices of the branch of yoga known as Hatha yoga. This technique alternates forceful, explosive, short exhalations with relaxed, soft, short inhalations.

How to do it…Place your open hand on your lower abdomen and make sure that your entire face and your neck and shoulders are relaxed. Quickly contract the muscles of your lower abdomen to push a strong burst of air out of your lungs and nose, and then immediately relax and allow your lungs to fill with air again. **When and for how long…**Try to repeat at least ten of these quick breath cycles at a rate of about one breath per second. Take a rest and then repeat. Finish by sitting quietly and allowing the breath to return to normal.

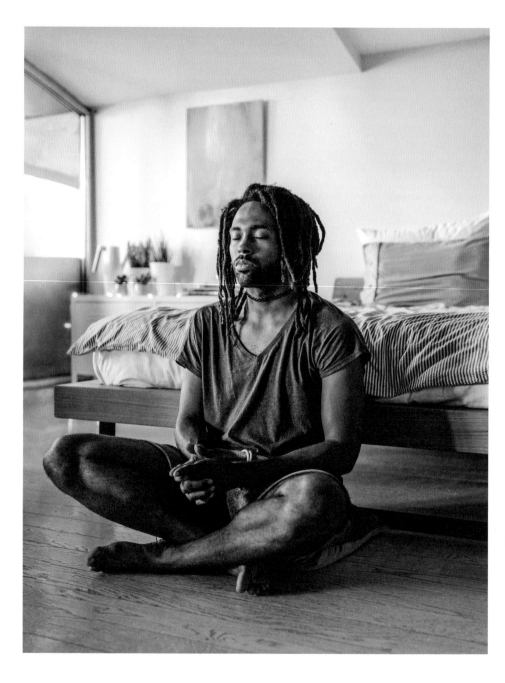

WHAT IS MEDITATION?

There is no single, fixed definition of meditation. Some would say that anything you do while consciously paying full attention to it qualifies as informal meditation, while formal meditation involves an intentional commitment of time, often sitting down to practise. The aim is to direct your attention away from external distractions for the benefit of mental focus and an increased sense of calm. With time, meditation allows you to sink below the chatter of your automatic thoughts and connect to a place of compassion toward yourself and others.

A WAY TO GAIN PERSPECTIVE

Among the many benefits of meditation are significantly reduced stress levels, improved cardiovascular health, better awareness and control of your emotions, and increased contentedness and productivity. Studies show, among other things, that people who meditate regularly need less sleep, and students perform significantly better in tests after meditating. Developing the ability to step away from your thoughts and see them in perspective helps you better understand and make sense of them.

It should be noted, however, that the practice does not work like an antidepressant or some happiness-inducing quick fix. On the contrary, for many people the first experience of meditation can be quite difficult – not only in a practical sense as they struggle to fend off distractions, but in an emotional way, too. When you're truly present, there's no escaping your emotions; if you are grieving or carrying around unresolved trauma, meditation will put it in the spotlight.

A SPACE FOR SELF-COMPASSION

How, then, can the very thing that highlights your inner struggle make you feel better? There's the neuroscientific explanation, which includes: a boost in the production of serotonin and dopamine (neurotransmitters responsible for our experience of wellbeing and happiness, lust and motivation); reduced cortisol (a naturally occurring steroid hormone, sometimes referred to as the "stress hormone") and stress levels; an increase in the brain's ability to organize and adapt; and a stimulated parasympathetic nervous system, making us feel calm and relaxed. And then there is the psychological knock-on effect: with improved hormonal balance and reduced stress levels, you gain empathy and perspective, feel more connected to yourself, and are able to deal with life's ups and downs in a calmer and more compassionate way.

It is hard for anxiety to thrive when you bring your attention to the present, refusing to rush into a spiral of worry. And it is easier to deal with troubles when you calm down and look at yourself in a nonjudgemental way.

WAYS TO MEDITATE

There are many different types of meditation. To find the one (or ones) that is right for you, you'll probably need to try out several. Here are eight of the best known and most popular.

1. TRANSCENDENTAL MEDITATION (TM)

Made famous by the Beatles, who met and were taught by Maharishi Mahesh Yogi in the 1960s, TM has a very specific goal: the state of enlightenment. When practising, you sit in the Lotus Posture, chant a mantra and focus on rising above negativity. If you want to learn, you should take a class or go on a retreat, as this is not something you can YouTube your way to – not least because you need to be given your own personal mantra.

2. BODY SCAN

Also known as progressive relaxation, this does just what the name suggests: allows you to scan your body for tension in order to notice and release it. You typically start at your feet and work your way up, or you can simply let the sensations guide you. It can be done on your own, without a guide, or you can follow a guided meditation through an app.

3. LOVING-KINDNESS MEDITATION

Also known as Metta Bhavana, this meditation helps you cultivate an attitude of compassion and love toward yourself and others. It involves deep breathing, opening up your mind to loving-kindness, and sending those same feelings out into the world. Through repetition, the sense of compassion generated can help combat feelings such as anger, inner conflict, resentment and frustration.

4. QI GONG

An old form of Chinese meditation (shown opposite) that uses a holistic system of breathing, movement and postures to circulate energy (*qi* means "life energy") through the body and promote balance. Learn the basics with a series of classes, then do your own home practice, enabling you to consciously rise and move into your day.

5. WALKING MEDITATION

In this form of meditation the sensation of walking is the focus. Many people find it slightly easier than some other forms of meditation since, when practising, they can pay attention to the outside world, such as sounds and wind. This meditation is best done outdoors. One grounding way to start the day may be to walk barefoot on grass, paying attention to nature as it wakes up.

6. GUIDED VISUALIZATION

A practice used to promote spiritual healing, stress relief and relaxation. Based on Buddha's belief that "the mind is everything and what you think you become", guided visualization focuses on one specific goal by imagining positive, relaxing experiences, which makes the body produce hormones and release chemicals to induce such feelings. While this is easy enough to try on your own, guided by a prerecorded audio track, it is a good idea to get some guidance by attending a class first.

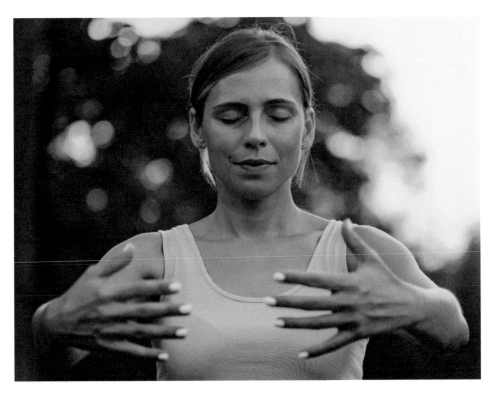

Nodding off?

Feeling sleepy during meditation is very common, and it's hardly surprising since meditation is done in the theta brain wave stage, during which we are in our subconscious mind, the body is asleep and we lose track of place and time, yet the mind is still awake and lucid. Prior to being able to achieve this state, when meditating we move from the beta brain-wave stage to the alpha stage, in which we relax and turn inward. It takes a lot of practice to move between these stages without nodding off, but be patient and kind to yourself. Opening a window when you sit down to meditate, making sure that you are well hydrated and getting a good night's sleep as often as you can may help.

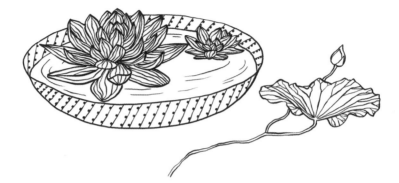

7. MINDFULNESS MEDITATION

While mindfulness is a theme in many kinds of meditation, Mindfulness Meditation has its roots in the Buddhist tradition and involves acknowledging and accepting any thoughts and sensations in a nonjudgemental way before letting them go and bringing your focus back to the present moment. This kind of meditation can be practised almost anywhere at any time and has been proved very useful in reducing anxiety and stress, as well as improving focus and memory.

8. MINDFULNESS OF BREATHING

During this breathing meditation, which is a form of Mindfulness Meditation (see above) you focus on your breath to become aware of the mind's tendency to wander. The simple practice of concentrating on the breath helps bring your full attention to the present moment and contributes to a sense of calm. You can practise on your own by repeatedly bringing your mind back to your breath, or your can follow the exercise on page 47.

Distracted?

Try meditating wearing a blindfold. The level of melatonin in the body goes down when we wake up and with daylight, but by wearing a blindfold when meditating first thing in the morning, you can keep the level high, which prevents you from entering an alert state.

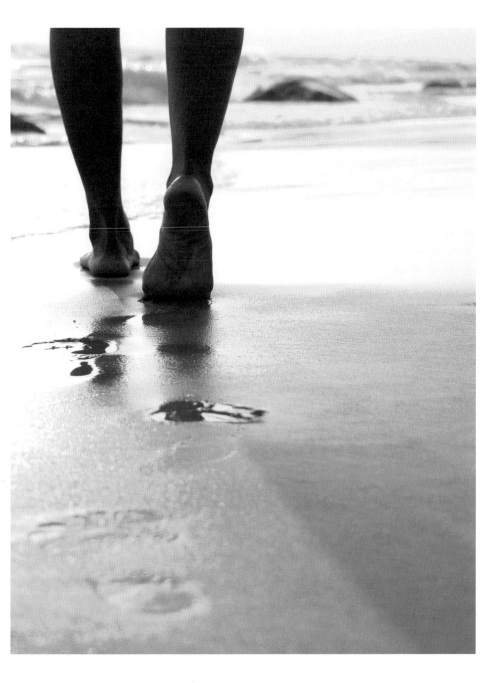

Tips for mastering meditation

1. Make sure you find a comfortable sitting position. You could sit on a chair, away from the chair back, with your back straight and your feet firmly on the floor. Or you could perhaps sit in a cross-legged position on a cushion or folded blanket on the floor, and your hands either in prayer position at the heart or resting gently on your thighs. If you have a yoga block, you could try the Seiza Posture, effectively kneeling but with the support of the block as a seat, and your hands resting in your lap.

2. Being nonjudgemental is central to meditation, so avoid thinking of a session as good or bad.

3. Always practise self-compassion, and don't set the bar too high. Mastering meditation takes time, and even after years of practice your mind will wander.

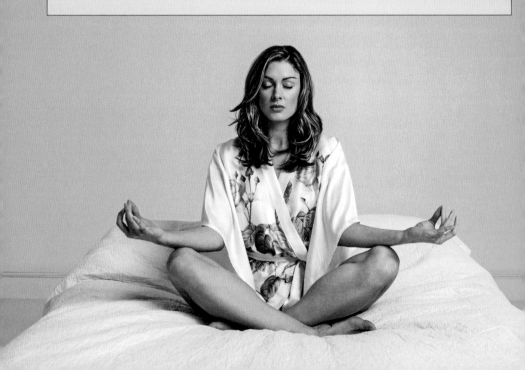

TRY MEDITATION

One of the huge advantages of meditation is that it can be completely free and entirely flexible: all you need is your own attention and you can take your practice with you wherever you go.

Having said that, there are a range of affordable and user-friendly apps available online. They can be hugely beneficial both in terms of reminding you of your daily session and in helping you understand the practice. One of the most popular is Headspace, developed by mindfulness teacher Andy Puddicombe and featuring hundreds of themed sessions of different lengths and kinds. Other popular meditation apps include Calm – featuring sleep stories and body programmes in addition to more than 100 guided meditations – and Stop, Breathe & Think, an emotional wellness platform for the under-25s.

AN EXERCISE: MINDFULNESS OF BREATHING MEDITATION

- Get comfortable, for example in an upright seated position, and set a timer on your alarm clock if you are giving yourself a digital-free space, or on your phone using a meditation app or the timer function. Start at 10 minutes and work up to as long as feels comfortable for you.

- Bring your attention to your breath, closing your mouth and allowing the breath to naturally flow in and out of your nose. Notice how it feels as the air enters your nose and how your lungs inflate and deflate. Imagine the breath travelling up and down the full length of your spine.

- Don't force your breathing – just notice it.

- Become aware of and acknowledge any thoughts, without judgment, as they enter your mind. Then let them go and bring your attention back to your breath.

- Remember to practise self-kindness. Your mind will wander – don't worry. Just keep bringing your attention back to your breath until the timer sounds.

IF YOU ONLY DO ONE THING...
Download Headspace, one of the most popular apps among secular meditators, on a free ten-day trial. This guided, no-frills meditation app is a great place to start.

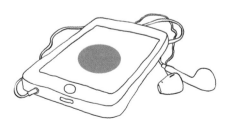

WHAT IS YOGA?

You could say that yoga is to the early 21st century what aerobics was to the 1990s, with classes at every gym and yoga pants for sale at every sports retailer. Trace its roots back to its origin, however, and you will find a practice that promotes far more than fitness and the ability to master a headstand.

The word yoga comes from the Sanskrit root *yuj* and is often described as a union of the mind and body. This says a lot about the original practice, which was as spiritual as it was physical, dating back to ancient Indian traditions. The poses we commonly refer to as yoga are, in fact, called *asana* – the physical postures that combine to allow us to reach a state of self-realization, where our automatic thoughts are no longer in charge and we are in control. This state, as well as the practice that enables this self-discovery and shift in awareness, is the true meaning of yoga.

THE SECRET OF YOGA

While the health benefits of the postures in yoga are many and well documented, the spiritual and cognitive journey is, in many ways, similar to that of meditation. Like meditation, yoga uses breath control to bring awareness of the distinction between our automatic thoughts and our being, to understand and accept that the thoughts we have in autopilot mode do not define and control us. In much the same way as in meditation and breath mastery, this awareness is the secret of yoga.

Nasal irrigation for improved breathing

Popular among yogis, nasal irrigation can take some getting used to, but is worth a try if you're a fan of *pranayama*.

Make a saline solution by dissolving ½ teaspoon salt in 125ml (4fl oz) boiled water. Once the water is lukewarm, stand bending forward with your head tilted to one side and use a neti pot to pour some solution into the upper nostril. The water will flush through your nasal passages and come out of the other nostril. Blow your nose and repeat on the other side.

"Yoga is the journey of the self, through the self, to the self."
— THE BHAGAVAD GITA

EARLY MORNING BED YOGA

Aisling Twomey is a banker by day and yogi by night. She teaches yoga under her brand Ióga by Aisling with the motto that yoga is for everyone. Morning yoga is a great way to start stretching and moving your body before you set about your day and, with these beginners' sequences, courtesy of Aisling, you don't even have to get out of bed.

Lots of people feel stiff and tight when they first wake up, so taking a few minutes to have a little stretch in bed can make all the difference. Be sure to move your bedclothes out of the way - no need to be neat about it, just make sure they're not an obstacle. (Of course, if you prefer, you can do these stretches on a mat on the floor.)

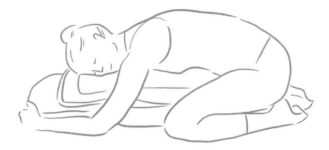

1. SUPPORTED BALASANA (CHILD'S POSE)
Grab two pillows (or several blankets) and stack them. Rest your chest and belly on the pillows, knees wide apart and feet tucked toward each other. Rest one side of your head on top of the pillows, close your eyes and bring your attention to your breath. Place your arms along the sides of the pillows or tuck them underneath like a big hug. Notice what it feels like to breathe, in and out, for a few minutes. Feel the slight stretch in your hips.

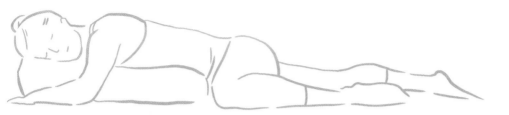

2. SUPPORTED ARDHA BHEKASANA (HALF FROG POSE)

Stay on your belly, removing one of the pillows so that you are lying on top of just one. Push one leg out to the side and bend your knee to form a 90-degree angle. Straighten the opposite leg down along the bed. Rest your head down, facing toward the bent leg. Bring the focus back to your breathing. After about ten breaths, repeat the posture on the other side, so that both sides feel balanced.

3. BHARMANASANA (TABLETOP POSITION)

Remove the pillows and push yourself up onto all fours, hands and knees on the bed. Your knees should be hip-width apart and your palms directly below your shoulders with the fingers pointing forward. Press down into your palms and knees, and lengthen your spine by pulling your shoulders away from your ears, with your tailbone and the crown of your head extending in opposite directions. Pay attention to your core muscles and pelvis to make sure that your back remains flat.

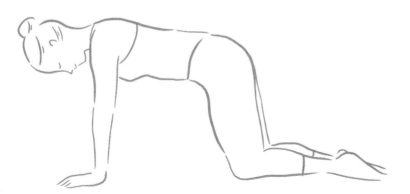

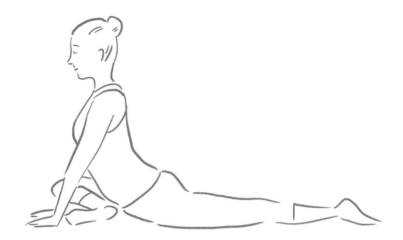

4. EKA PADA RAJAKAPOTASANA (PIGEON POSE)

From the *Bharmanasana* Position, push your right leg forward so that the knee is behind your right wrist, the shin on a diagonal and the heel pointing to your left hipbone. Stretch your left leg out behind you. Keep your hands down on the bed or, if you want to deepen the stretch, wriggle into it some more, fold forward and rest your head on your hands. After about ten breaths, come back to *Bharmanasana*, swap your legs around and repeat on the other side.

5. SUPTA BADDHA KONASANA (RECLINED BOUND ANGLE POSE)

Flip over and lie flat on your back. Bring the soles of your feet together with your legs bent. If your knees don't reach right down to the bed, pop a pillow underneath each one; fold the pillows if you need to. This one is all about good support, so you can add another pillow under your head if you want to. Feel free to take up space: reach your arms out to the sides with the palms facing up toward the sky. Close your eyes and breathe deeply.

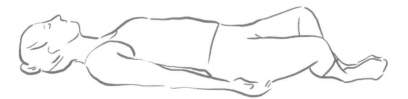

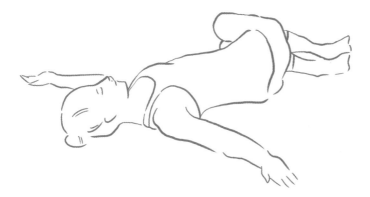

6. SUPPORTED RECLINED TWIST

Still on your back, bring the soles of your feet to the bed, knees pointing up. Let both legs fall to the left. Slip a pillow between your thighs if it helps. Try to keep your upper back flat on the bed – you're trying to achieve a slight twist in your body. Extend your arms out to the sides at shoulder level, with the palms of your hands facing up, and enjoy the twist down the side of your body for a few breaths. Keep your head centred, nose pointing up to the ceiling and eyes closed, or turn your head slightly to face to the right. When you're ready to swap sides, carefully bring your legs back up and rest the soles of your feet on the bed for a second, before dropping your legs, and turning your head, to the other side.

7. FULL BODY STRETCH

Once you are done with your morning yoga, lie flat on your back with plenty of space above you. Inhale deeply and reach your arms out overhead. Have a long, luxurious stretch and really commit to it; feel the stretch from the very tops of your fingers to the very tips of your toes. As you exhale, fold your knees in toward your chest and wrap your arms around your legs. Give yourself a little hug.

Enjoy a moment of rest before you get up; set an intention (see page 57) for the day ahead or have a moment of gratitude (see page 96). Maybe enjoy some herbal tea for a last few minutes of relaxation.

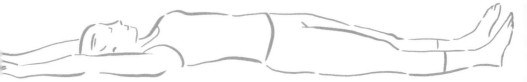

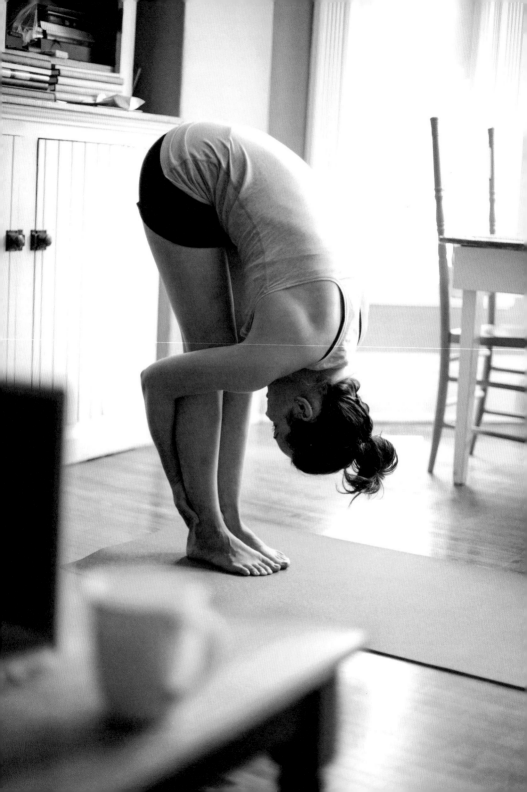

TIPS AND RESOURCES FOR MORNING YOGIS

Give yourself time. Like meditation, yoga is a practice that gets better with time, and you might feel far from that state of self-realization the first time you try it. But as you figure out the poses and are able to go deeper into the stretches without having to pay too much attention to every word your instructor says, you will feel stronger and more relaxed. Be patient and don't aim for perfection.

Ignore the Instagram culture and the fancy yoga pants. Wear whatever you feel comfortable in and don't focus too much on the Flying Pigeons and flat abs. You'll get there one day if you want to. Try to stay present on the mat, not on social media.

RESOURCES FOR BEGINNERS

Online sessions…Adriene Mishler of Yoga with Adriene has won countless awards for her series of video sessions, including everything from 30-day plans to tutorials for each individual pose. There are endless programmes for yogis of all levels. Try a few sessions free of charge on YouTube, or sign up and become part of her growing community.

Tutorials and more…Rachel Brathen, aka Yoga Girl, is another popular online facilitator, whose community platform, oneOeight, offers tutorials, training programmes, counselling and peer-to-peer support.

Community spirit…If you have a yoga hub nearby, a face-to-face community can be priceless. Even if you choose to make your yoga a solo morning thing, attending some sessions is likely to be worthwhile because you'll get some expert advice on improving your alignment within postures.

WHAT YOU NEED

- A yoga mat is an affordable investment that is worth its weight in gold if you think you'll stick with the practice. I've done yoga on decking and hardwood floors, and it's just not the same.

- Some people like a yoga block for adding support to certain poses, but you don't *need* one – a thick book works just fine, at least in the beginning.

- Yoga leggings are great, but you don't necessarily need them. Just avoid floaty garments that you'll get tangled up in. Don't wear socks – they'll make you feel less stable and could even make you slip, in addition to the fact that they take away from your connection with the ground and can therefore make it harder to spread your toes for full support.

WHO IS YOGA FOR?

Yoga is perfect for those who want some mental space and to work on that awareness, but who also enjoy a raised pulse and a gentle workout. You don't have to be fit when you begin – just start where you are and figure it out at your own pace.

Yoga suits those who perhaps like the idea of meditation but struggle with being focused. You can't do yoga without being fully present: it's very difficult to be mentally composing an email while focusing on balancing one-legged in *Vrksasana* (Tree Pose).

Some styles of yoga may suit you better than others. If you are looking for dynamic movement and want to raise your pulse quickly, try Ashtanga yoga. Look to Iyengar yoga for precision and focus on alignment, or try Yin yoga if you want a slower, more meditative practice.

Although club memberships are often pricey, you can pretty much keep up yoga practice even if you're broke, as you can do it at home. The added bonus is that you can take it with you wherever you go – to the hotel room on a work trip or to the beach on holidays.

IF YOU ONLY DO ONE THING...

Try Yoga with Adriene's Yoga for Beginners series. I know so many people who started here and never looked back, so this will tell you whether you've found your thing or not.

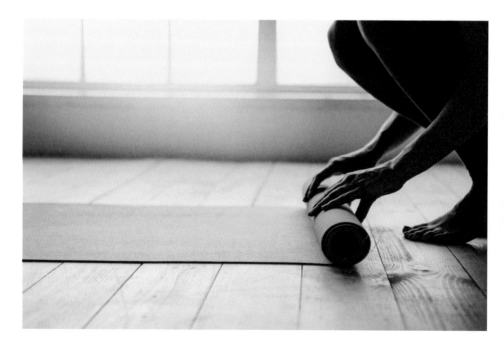

A TOOLKIT

For meditators, yogis and other self-discoverers
there are a number of resources you can tap
into to make the most of your discipline.

INTENTIONS

The dictionary definition of an intention is "an act or instance of determining mentally upon some action or result". Intentions are often used in self-care and productivity practices as a commitment to a mental state or way of being that we aspire to. Most people start an intention with "My intention is to…", and then it can be anything from "…be positive in all my interactions with colleagues" to "…act with integrity according to my values". There are many ways to work with intentions, from writing them down and reviewing them every day to saying them out loud at the end of a meditation session. Typically, a good bit of time, planning and self-examination go into finding the intentions that are right at any given point, and they can then be used for weeks or months before they are replaced.

AFFIRMATIONS

While intentions look to the future, whether for the day or month ahead, an affirmation is a statement about something that is true at the present moment – and something that you want to be true. Affirmations usually start with "I am…" and can declare strength, honesty, focus or anything in between – for instance, "I am calm" when facing a daunting task; "I am at peace" when working on letting go of destructive habits or thoughts; or "I am strong" when preparing for a tough challenge.

Some people prefer intentions over affirmations as they are more authentic and don't brush over any feelings of doubt or fear you may be experiencing right now. Others find that affirmations are more effective as they are to the point and immediate.

MIND MOVIE

A powerful tool, the mind movie is a short video depicting your idea of the perfect life, which allows you, in effect, to experience it in the present moment. It can contain images of beautiful places, things that inspire you or pictures of you doing what you love, all with your favourite uplifting track in the background and perhaps an affirmation or two. There are countless apps and online widgets to help you create your mind movie.

A toolkit tip

End a meditation or yoga session by watching your mind movie. You will be in a calm, receptive state of mind and really able to internalize your goals and affirmations before you go about your day.

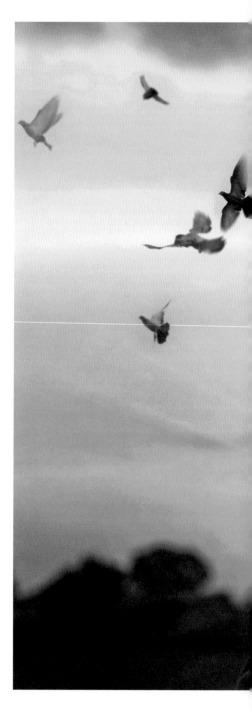

VISION BOARD

Hugely popular, perhaps because they combine the benefits of intentions and mind movies with a creative session – think collage meets scrapbook – vision boards contain pictures cut out of magazines, photographs and drawings and motivational words. Together they represent your vision for the road ahead or capture a mood you hope to experience in the coming weeks or season. It should get a prominent spot in a reasonably private part of your home, perhaps at your home altar (see page 165), if you have one.

PRAYER

If you have a religious faith, you may have read the descriptions on this and the previous page and thought to yourself that this is what prayer is for. This is, of course, highly individual: it depends on your religious beliefs whether you engage in prayer at all and, if so, how you do it. Perhaps you pray for guidance and strength at a difficult time or ask for the blessing of something you're hoping to do or achieve. If prayer provides you with hope and vitality, it may be the only tool you need.

"First thing
every morning
before you arise
say out loud,
'I believe,'
three times."
— OVID

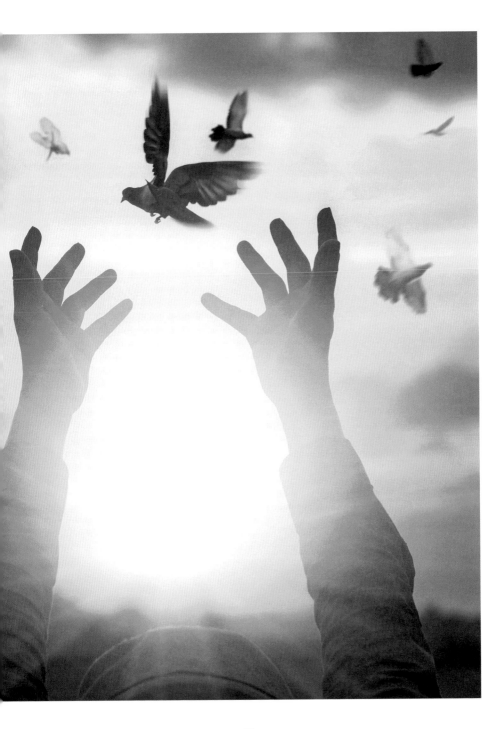

BREATHE – SUGGESTED RITUALS

Breathe your way to a calm, focused start

Use your breath as a vehicle for stretching out the kinks in your body and warming it up, combining the benefits of mindfulness with the goodness of oxygen. By tweaking one of these suggested rituals to suit your situation, you can start your day feeling fully present - in both body and mind.

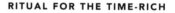

RITUAL FOR THE TIME-POOR

– Rise early.

– Complete four repetitions of 4-7-8 breathing (see page 38) as you wait for the kettle to boil.

– Prepare and drink a glass of warm lemon water (see page 110).

– Take a shower and get dressed.

– Grab a boiled egg and a handful of nuts for breakfast on the go (see page 115).

– If you walk to work, or indeed to the bus stop or train station, practise a walking meditation (see page 42).

RITUAL FOR THE TIME-RICH

– Rise before dawn.

– Stretch out the body with a bed yoga routine (see page 50).

– Get comfortable on the balcony, in your garden or at an open window, with a blanket if it's cold, and enjoy a cup of herbal tea as you watch the sun rise (see page 151).

– Take a bath with essential oils and complete a body scan meditation (see page 42) as you soak.

– Enjoy a bowl of overnight oats with added fresh berries (see page 115) before you leave the house or get started with work.

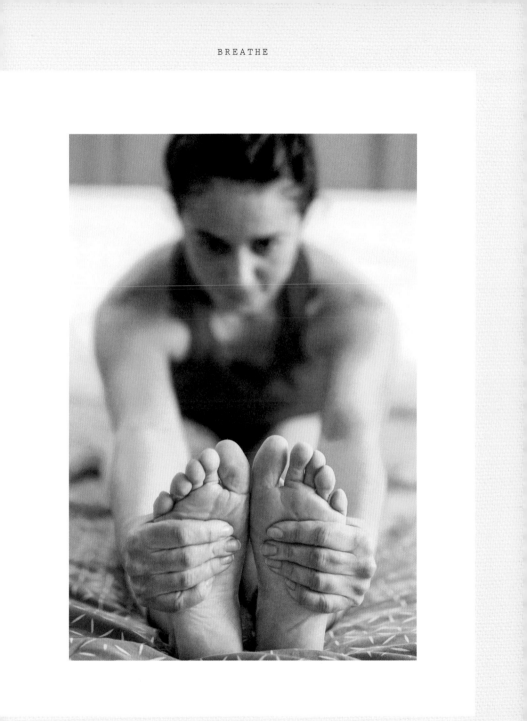

"Methinks that the moment
my legs began to move,
my thoughts began to flow."
— HENRY DAVID THOREAU

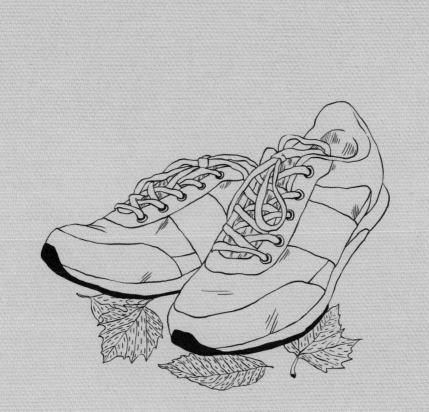

CHAPTER 3

AWAKEN

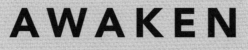

Active workout rituals

WHAT HAPPENS WHEN YOU EXERCISE?

Every time I'm back from a run, I am filled with the same feeling: a sort of blissful ecstasy, and disbelief that the key to happiness can be so simple. I want to tell the world to run, run, run. Such is the joy of what they call the "runner's high" - in neuroscientific terms, a release of endorphins. These neurotransmitters interact with the receptors in your brain that reduce your perception of pain, but endorphins are also known to contribute to a surge of positivity and euphoria.

"RUNNER'S HIGH" EXPLAINED

This high is not exclusive to runners; it is served up alongside all kinds of exercise and workouts. And accompanying this very welcome dose of endorphins comes an abundance of other generous neurotransmitters, such as serotonin, dopamine and oxytocin – all boosting happiness, but connected to, respectively, a sense of meaning and importance, desire and drive, trust and intimacy.

There are also beneficial knock-on effects of exercise, including: reduced stress, anxiety and depression; greatly improved sleep; a boost in self-esteem; improved communication and cognitive skills; and a brain better able to develop new neural pathways. Your brain starts to work at optimum capacity, which makes your nerve cells multiply and grow stronger; new blood vessels form; your blood pressure drops; and your resting heart rate decreases.

HOW MUCH AND HOW OFTEN?

From your brain to your gut and right through your joints and bones, exercise is good for you – and guess what? Doing a little every day contributes more to your general health and wellbeing than two or three longer weekly sessions.

Just 20 minutes is enough to change the way the brain processes information and memories. Then the benefits multiply over time: already after your first session, your brain function will improve; after a week of regular exercise, you will feel your energy levels increase and your cells will start to benefit; one month in, you'll have increased your muscle mass and your metabolism; after six months, your heart will be bigger and stronger; and for every day of exercise, your mental health benefits more and more.

"A feeble body
weakens the mind."
— JEAN-JACQUES ROUSSEAU

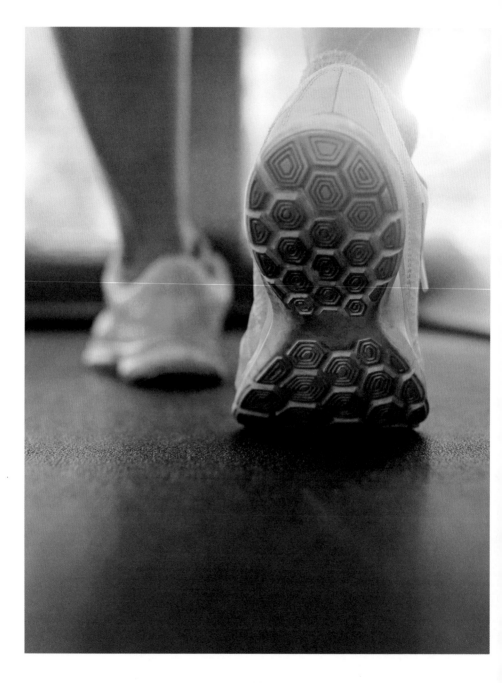

WHY WORK OUT IN THE MORNING?

Preference aside, is there any reason why morning exercise is particularly good for you?

BOOSTING YOUR GET GO

Studies have shown that morning workouts are likely to contribute to a good night's sleep. I know when I've been riding that runner's high too late at night, as I'm unable to wind down because of the ecstasy. A morning workout is also great for getting your metabolism going – and, perhaps the most convincing argument of all, people who exercise in the morning are more inclined to keep it up. Unsurprisingly, you're more likely to find that other things get in the way when you've planned to go for a run at night – sometimes, ironically, simply because you never got that energy boost in the morning and you're just too tired.

BEING ONE STEP AHEAD

Many people seem to be of the "get it out of the way" school of thought, which is perhaps not the mindset you want to aim for, but is understandable nonetheless. And by exercising first thing, you also pave the way for a whole range of other benefits, as a result of your increased energy throughout the day and a positive start thanks to those endorphins and all that serotonin. Greeting the world in its most serene state is a lovely, grounding experience. By doing so with a workout session you get to start the day knowing that you have already achieved something _and_ been kind to yourself. According to a Bristol University study, your concentration levels at work may be up by as much as 21 percent, too, if you exercise in the morning, while your productivity can skyrocket by 41 percent and your risk of burnout goes right down.

AIDING ALL-ROUND SELF-DISCIPLINE

Think of your morning workout session as an intention to start the day as you mean to go on. You'll then be able to understand how, for many, carrots seem a more appealing mid-morning snack than a slice of cake. The self-discipline tends to spill into other aspects of your life, and that morning promise to take care of your body can grow into a day-long commitment to being good and kind to yourself.

> "An early morning walk is a blessing for the whole day."
> — HENRY DAVID THOREAU

MORNING WORKOUT INSPIRATION

---

*Running at daybreak tends to be addictive, but getting out
the door on a wet winter's morning can be incredibly difficult,
so you might want to combine it with other forms of exercise.
A weights workout can give you a lovely boost within the comfort
of your own home, but perhaps your housemates disapprove of that
upbeat music at 6am. What works for you depends on everything
from preference to circumstance - but rest assured that there
is no shortage of options. Here are just a few of them...*

RUNNING

Incredible mental and physical health benefits aside, much of the beauty of running lies in its simplicity. In many ways, this is brain work: as you build up stamina, it is you against your brain. If you can figure out how to stay motivated and mentally strong, you will quickly notice the benefits and are likely to get the bug. You can do it anywhere, and the only thing you really need is a pair of running shoes – unless, of course, you want to hop on the barefoot running trend. In recent years, perhaps thanks to the growing popularity of running, many workplaces have installed shower facilities on site. What could be easier than packing your breakfast and hopping straight into your running shoes when you wake up, to run all the way to your desk?

POWER WALKING

While you need to work up a good pace to make sure that your heart gets the workout it needs, a brisk walk can bring you all the benefits of running without that same initial mental challenge. Perhaps you're injured

> ### Tip for novice runners
>
> Create an upbeat playlist of tracks you like. Alternate brisk walking for one song with running or jogging for one song. Start and end with walking, and try to keep going for 25 minutes. As you start to feel fitter and stronger, you can run for two tracks at a time.

or have health complications that mean you can't run, or you commute to work and can't incorporate a run into your journey, or you want to walk your dog, or maybe you just love walking. For an increased upper-body workout and cardiovascular benefits, you

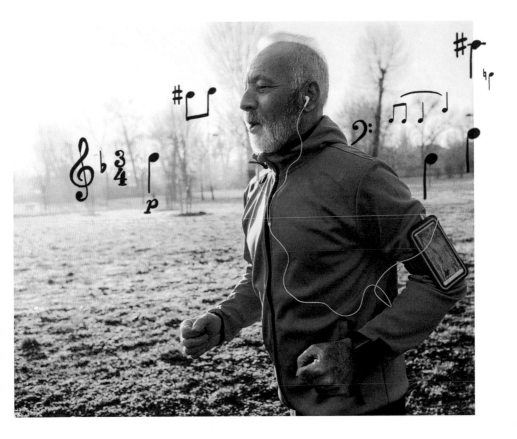

could buy a pair of Nordic walking poles. Find a good podcast for added inspiration, and step confidently and powerfully into your day.

KETTLEBELLS

Combining both strength and cardiovascular exercise, kettlebells offer a best-of-both-worlds fix, targeting muscles all the way from your head to your toes, including some you might easily overlook in a traditional workout session. With endless tutorials available free of charge online, you can find exactly the programme that suits you.

GYM AND GROUP TRAINING

A gym has the benefit of a community of people cheering each other on and holding each other to account. You're greeted with a smile as you walk through the door every morning, and there are people to share your progress with. There will be a wide range of equipment and classes so you can tailor your exercise to your own needs. Gym membership isn't cheap, but for some the cost is itself a source of motivation, almost like a contract with yourself that you are going to get value out of it in the form of improved health.

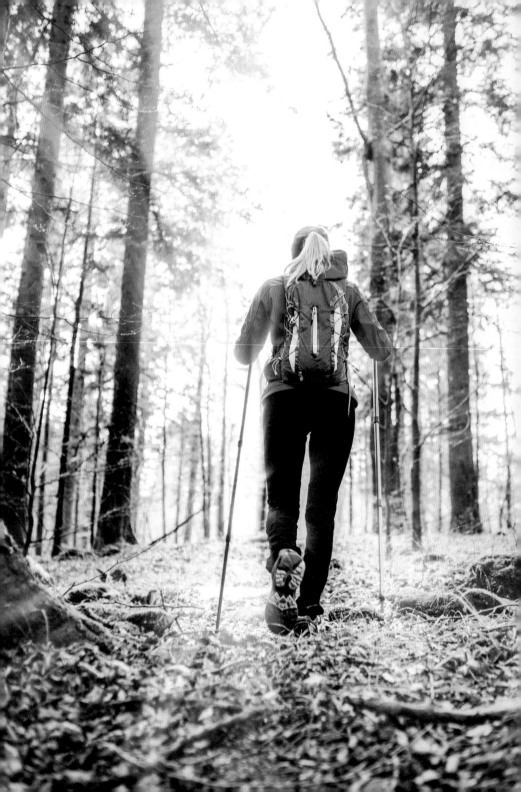

A PHYSIOTHERAPIST
ON MORNING EXERCISE

Sara Pettersson is a physiotherapist and exercise enthusiast who has been working out and playing sports her entire life. Here, she shares her top tips for effective but sensible morning exercise, as well as some advice on how to stay motivated.

THINGS TO CONSIDER

"When the body has been inactive for hours, it's important to move gently and slowly at first, just to wake up joint and muscle structures and the body as a whole. No quick, forced movements in the beginning – but once you warm up, you can go ahead and push yourself a little harder."

MOTIVATIONAL TIPS FOR BEGINNERS

"Don't make it too complicated. Don't set the bar too high, but make sure that you set clear goals that feel achievable yet challenging – that's important for the motivation.

"If in doubt, ask someone in the know, and maybe find a workout buddy so that you can take turns to motivate and cheer each other on when the going gets tough."

WHY EXERCISE IN THE MORNING?

"I love running in the morning if I've had a good night's sleep – it's amazing! To greet the day when it's so calm and peaceful, before all the traffic and people speed things up; to get to start the day with that wonderful feeling, in both the body and the mind, is so satisfying and has such positive benefits for your mood and the energy you'll have for other activities throughout the day. And, of course, there's always the practical benefit of getting your workout done in the morning: then the rest of the day is left for other things."

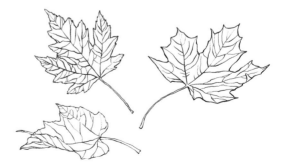

FULL-BODY HOME WORKOUT

Courtesy of physiotherapist Sara Pettersson (see page 71), here is a morning workout programme to get you started. Aim to go gently but keep a steady pace, and repeat the full set three times. If you are a beginner, take it easy, and perhaps start with two rounds as you build up strength.

Tips for a mindful workout

1. Watch out for any tension in the body. As a starting point, be mindful of your hips and core and keep your lower back supported. Relax your forehead and drop your shoulders.

2. Don't forget to breathe. Holding your breath during tough exercises is a common mistake, but you need to keep breathing to make sure that your muscles get the oxygen they need. The best thing to do is to breathe through your mouth with a relaxed jaw, mouth slightly open and lips not pursed.

3. It's always nice to end a workout session with a moment of mindfulness, either seated with your legs crossed and eyes closed or standing with your hands together in Prayer Pose at your heart, bringing your chin to the chest.

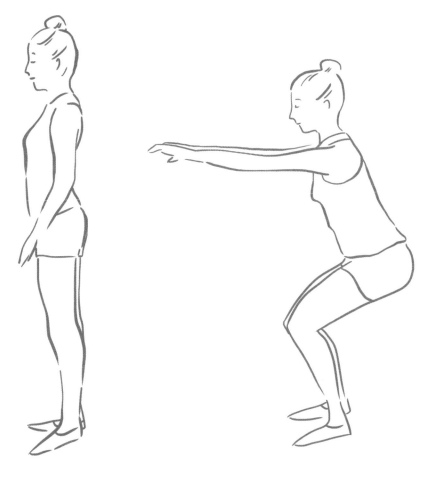

1. SQUATS

Stand with your feet hip-width apart, with the
toes pointing to five past eleven. Bend your
knees and squat down, as if you were going
to sit on a chair. Make sure that your knees
are positioned directly above your feet, then
straighten up to standing. Repeat 15 times.

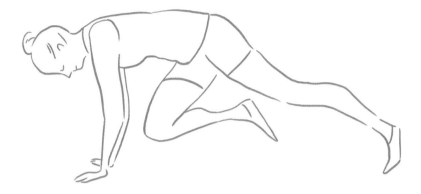

2. MOUNTAIN CLIMBER

Start in a Plank Pose, in which your body rests horizontally like a straight board, with your hands on the ground directly below your shoulders, your arms straight and your toes on the floor. Use your core muscles to keep your body in a straight line. Bend one knee up toward your chest, raising your buttocks slightly, and then straighten the leg again. Swap legs. Repeat 15 times per leg.

3. PRONE COBRA

Lie down on your belly with your arms along your sides and the backs of your hands resting on the floor. Raise your head and back a little bit while twisting your arms so that the backs of your hands point upward. Squeeze your shoulder blades together. Release back to the floor. Repeat 15 times.

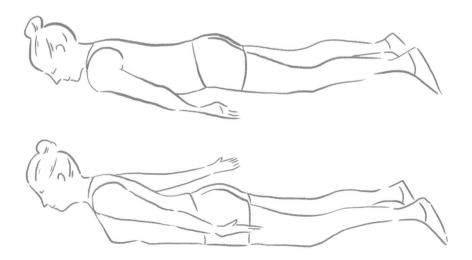

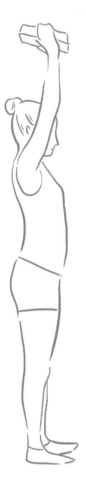

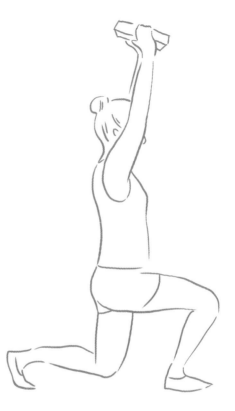

4. LUNGES

Stand with your feet together. Hold a large book or something similar above your head with your arms straight. Step your right foot forward in a lunge (a big step forward, bending the right knee, lowering the body and dropping the left knee straight down) – avoid pushing the right knee forward further than the right foot. Rise back up in a controlled motion to standing with your feet together. Swap legs. Repeat 15 times per leg.

5. PELVIC LIFT

Lie on your back. Bend both knees and, with your feet flat on the floor, lift your hips so that your body forms a straight line from shoulder to knee. Stretch one leg out while stabilizing your hip and torso, and hold the position for 3 seconds. Return to the starting position before swapping legs. Repeat 15 times per leg.

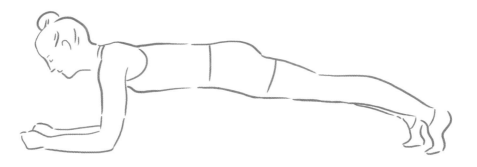

6. FOREARM PLANK

Get into the Forearm Plank Pose (similar to the Plank described under Mountain Climber on page 74, but with your arms bent so that you rest on your elbows, which should be directly below your shoulders). Your forearms should be parallel to your body and your legs straight, with your toes on the floor. Aim for a straight line from the top of your head through your neck and spine, through your hips, buttocks and legs – and don't let your head drop. Hold for 15 seconds.

7. FOREARM SIDE PLANK

Change into Forearm Side Plank by flipping your feet so that one rests on top of the other, and you are resting on your right elbow, with it directly below your right shoulder. Place your left hand on your left hip. Now lift your body, holding yourself up on the right arm and the side of your right foot, keeping your hips lifted and your body in a straight line. Hold for 15 seconds. Drop to the ground, flip to the other side, and repeat.

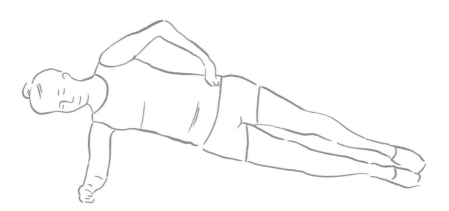

THE HEALING
POWERS OF WATER

---

*Water immersion and swimming have had deeply loyal fans for a
long time and seem to keep winning over devotees. While some may
simply be looking for a new way to feel refreshed and renewed,
there are others who use it to help deal with grief or burnout.
Some people meet in groups for daily dips, while others just
take the opportunity to swim whenever and wherever they can,
but what all of them have in common is an enthusiasm for
the incredibly comforting, healing powers of water.*

HYDROTHERAPY

Since ancient times, hydrotherapy has
been employed to treat ailments. Being
submerged in water can provide a sense
of calm as a result of sensory information
being dulled. It is believed that the pressure
of water against one's chest boosts the flow of
blood to the brain, and studies have shown
that flotation tank therapy (time spent in body-
temperature water with so much salt that the
body floats, belly up, without any effort) helps
relieve symptoms of chronic stress.

MINDFUL EXERCISE

When you exercise in water, you reap all the
benefits of the exercise itself while being held
by the water. This has a range of advantages,
particularly if you are recovering from injury
or for other reasons need to be mindful of
the strain you put on your body. Recreational
swimming takes some of the impact stress off
your body as you work on endurance, fitness
and heart and lung health, and it strengthens

almost all the muscles. Moreover, swimming
has a relaxing, calming effect and helps
improve posture, flexibility and coordination.

Opinion is divided as to whether or not
your body needs a day of rest after strenuous
exercise, but with swimming you don't need
to worry. Even with higher-intensity swimming,
the wear and tear on the body is not the
same – some people even use swimming
as the gentle option for their rest day.

GETTING STARTED WITH SWIMMING

Live right by the sea? Then your mood-
boosting, Instagram-friendly morning ritual
is a no-brainer. Not lucky enough to live in the
Tropics? Make sure you read the tips for cold
water swimming on pages 152–3. Alternatively,
there's nothing wrong with a membership at
your local pool, where the water will no doubt
be warmer. Plus, you are more likely to benefit
from the camaraderie of fellow morning
swimmers than if braving the waves alone.

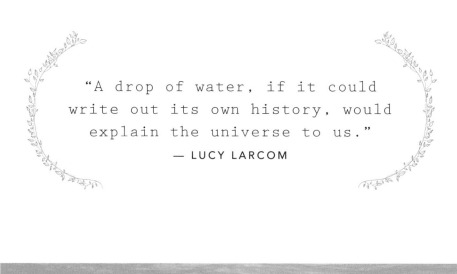

"A drop of water, if it could
write out its own history, would
explain the universe to us."
— LUCY LARCOM

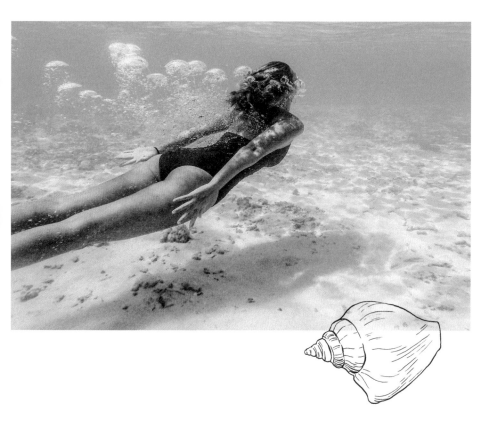

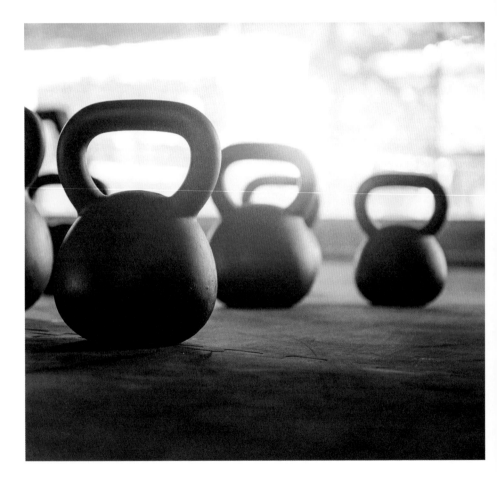

TIPS AND TOOLS FOR MORNING WORKOUTS

Don't let a tight budget or a lack of previous experience and an already established fitness regime hold you back. Even newbies can fall head over heels for a mini morning jog ritual.

WHAT YOU NEED

With a decent pair of running shoes and shorts or comfortable leggings, you can get through most workout regimes. A smartphone app for tracking your run or giving you exercise cues takes things straight to the next level. Perhaps hold off on the gym membership until you've proved to yourself that you're committed to your new morning routine. Once you know you're sticking to it, you can look at wearable wireless trackers of different kinds, which help you keep track of everything from your heart rate and number of calories burned to floors climbed, and perhaps upgrade your running shoes or invest in different weights.

IF YOU ONLY DO ONE THING...

Try it once. Exercise can feel quite different in the morning from a work-energy-fuelled evening gym session. Go for a morning jog or swim, or try a workout session, just to see how you feel.

Tips for maintaining motivation

There will be days when putting on the gym gear is a struggle. Prepare for those days by giving yourself a challenge or a treat: register for a race that you have to train for, create a kilometres-per-week challenge among friends, or promise yourself a spa experience after a month of morning exercise.

If sharing the ups and downs of a workout routine helps you stay motivated, join a training group on social media or find one of the many exercise challenge hashtags that are doing the rounds on Instagram, such as the 30-day #plankchallenge.

AWAKEN – SUGGESTED RITUALS

Find your flow with activity and movement

With or without fresh air, starting your day by increasing your pulse rate and even breaking into a sweat can set you up for success and sustained energy levels throughout the day. Take inspiration from one of these rituals, adapt it to your needs and enjoy feeling strong and alive.

RITUAL FOR THE TIME-POOR

– The evening before, get prepped for a run to work by ensuring you have a change of clothes – and underwear – at the office, or your sports backpack packed accordingly.

– Get straight into your running gear when you wake up.

– If fasted workouts are not for you, have a banana or simply blitz together a green smoothie (see page 114) for an energy boost; alternatively, leave breaking the fast for later (see pages 108, 121 and the exercise tip on page 122).

– Run or jog to work (see page 68).

– Shower and dress at work, and you're all set for the day ahead.

RITUAL FOR THE TIME-RICH

– Rise early.

– Sitting on the edge of the bed or in a comfortable seat of your choice, take a moment to pay attention to your breath for a few minutes and set an intention for the day ahead (see page 57).

– Do the full-body home workout (see page 72), completing three rounds of all exercises.

– Take an ice-cold shower (see page 135).

– Have breakfast while reviewing your goals for the day ahead (see page 114).

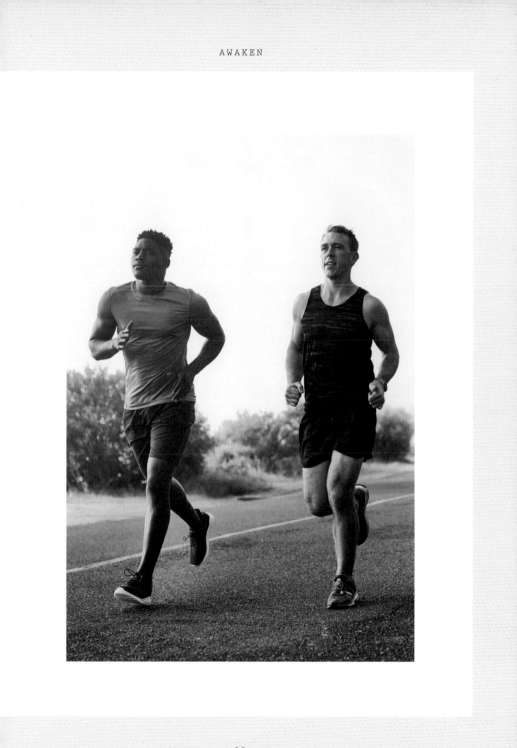

"...there are a thousand thoughts
lying within a man that he does
not know till he takes up the
pen to write."

— WILLIAM MAKEPEACE THACKERAY

CHAPTER 4

FOCUS

Rituals for a clear mind

BRAIN TRAINING

---

*The brain is not a muscle, but it behaves a lot like one.
Crucially, it can be trained as though it were a muscle. Your
brain feels tired when you've learned something new, rather like
your muscles hurting after a tough workout, but as you keep
challenging your brain, it develops and becomes more agile.*

LEARNING POSITIVITY

The brain has something of a hang-up when it comes to negative experiences – they tend to stick. It's called a negativity bias and it actually makes a lot of sense: the brain is programmed to protect us, so it is constantly on the lookout for threats and potential problems. Positivity, meanwhile, is perfectly safe and therefore goes almost unnoticed.

The good news is that we can counteract a negativity bias, thanks to the plasticity of the brain and an awareness that, in fact, we do need positivity. Enter meditation (see page 41) and different kinds of journalling (see page 89). Set goals, and you will feel calmer; make plans, and you will begin to relax; think about the good things in life, and your brain will slowly but surely start to pay attention.

IT'S NEVER TOO LATE

Our experiences mould and reprogramme the brain on a continuous basis. It might seem unfair that, in terms of brain-programming, people who grow up in a calm, safe and happy environment have an automatic advantage over those who experienced a lot of fear and uncertainty during their childhood, but at least the door is open and it's never too late to improve the situation.

Meditation will encourage you to bring your awareness to the present moment instead of the past or the future. Journalling, goal setting and visualization will help you to be selective as well as bring awareness to the things in your life that are going well – in addition to shedding light on the doors of opportunity. So it's time to plan for some brain training every morning.

"The brain is wider
than the sky."
— EMILY DICKINSON

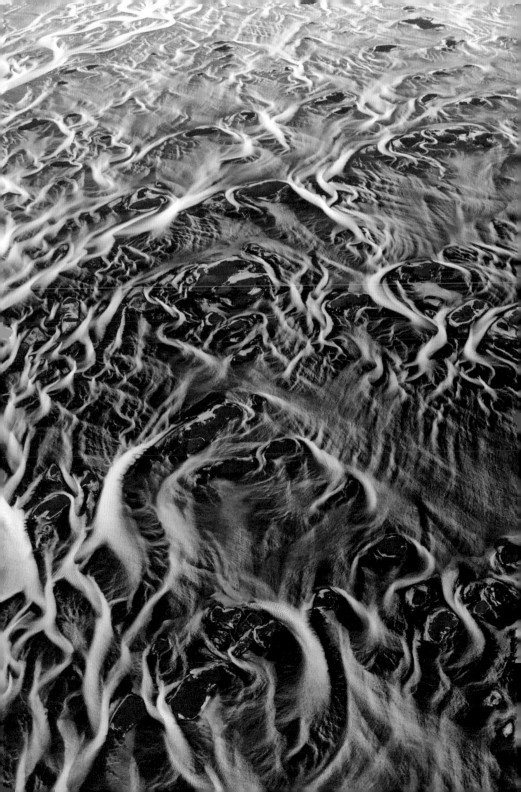

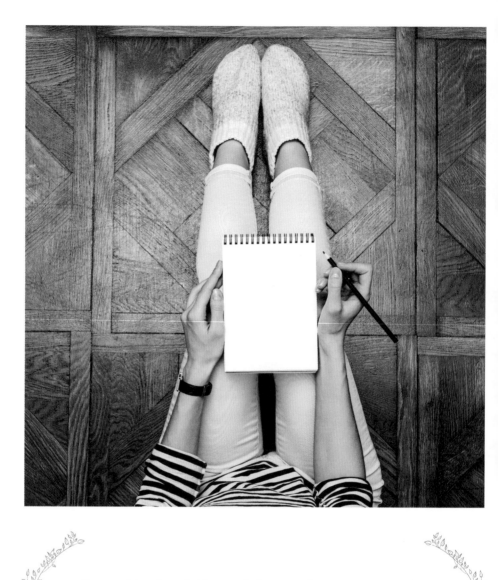

"...it is like whispering to one's self and listening at the same time."
— MINA MURRAY IN BRAM STOKER'S *DRACULA*

THE PROMISE OF A BLANK PAGE

Many people describe their morning ritual as a way to take control of their day. A blank page is a powerful symbol of that: a space to fill, full of promise, free from constriction and restraint. As you fill the page with gratitude, intentions and goals, you free up space in your mind.

That said, one type of journalling can be very different from the next. While writing has proved an effective tool in the field of positive psychology, it is also at the top of the list for productivity gurus and creative types alike. Here are some of the most commonly used writing tools of early risers.

GOAL SETTING

There are as many ways of working with goal setting as there are people setting goals but, simply speaking, this is about clarity and focus. Anything that doesn't get you closer to the goal is a distraction and probably a waste of time. The idea is that being conscious of your dreams and direction helps you to behave and prioritize accordingly. Read more on page 99.

MORNING PAGES

Part of the toolkit in the poet, playwright and filmmaker Julia Cameron's hugely popular book *The Artist's Way*, the morning pages are simply three pages of stream-of-consciousness writing done first thing every morning, free from rules, goals and audiences. Countless writers and other creatives around the world swear by the habit as a way of clearing the head and making room for creativity.

TO-DO LISTS

Spending time in the morning looking over your to-do list and prioritizing tasks is nothing new – but perhaps it remains popular simply because it is tried and tested. Putting pen to paper to decide on your focus before you start your day helps you get back to what matters. Moreover, and crucially, the knowledge that all the important tasks are on the list provides a kind of mental space and peace of mind that are otherwise hard to come by.

"BUJO"

Perhaps the newest and most talked-about journalling practice is bullet journalling, often lovingly referred to by devotees as BuJo. This is more advanced than many of the other methods, involving deeply considered layouts and grids, and appealing to those who have a penchant for design elements such as lettering. Visual fanciness aside, people find bullet journalling invaluable when it comes to planning ahead, getting a good overview and staying on top of daily tasks and chores.

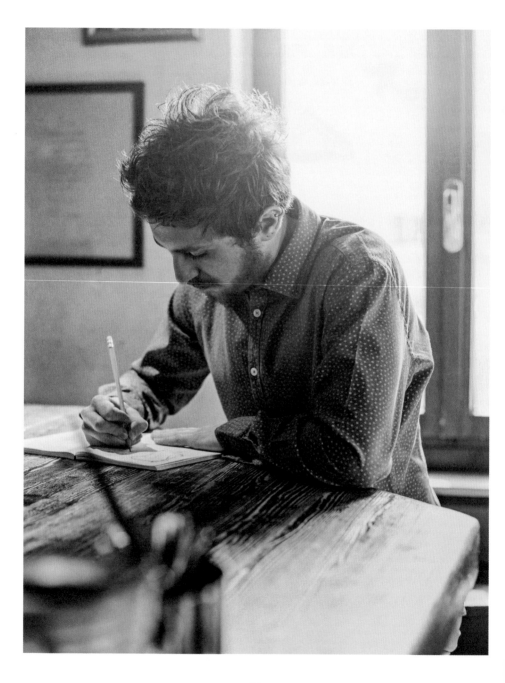

RECORDING GRATITUDE

Remember that car game played on long journeys where whoever counts ten yellow cars first wins? Imagine if someone asked how many blue cars you had seen. You wouldn't be able to say, because you would have been too busy focusing on yellow.

That may sound overly simplistic but, in fact, it's not all that far-fetched. When our minds are preoccupied by chores and worries, it's easy to forget about much of what's right in front of us – all the things we take for granted. That's not necessarily a failure on our part, but once we become aware of it we can use it to our advantage and retrain our brains to focus on the goodness in life.

ARE YOU HAPPIER THAN YOU THINK?

In the same way as antidepressants boost neurotransmitters such as dopamine and serotonin, which regulate everything from motivation to emotional and cognitive functions and, simply speaking, contribute to our sense of wellbeing, so, too, does thinking about the things in life that you are grateful for. Far from fooling your brain into thinking you're happy, the practice of gratitude journalling allows you to see that you already *are* happy.

GO ON, JUST THREE THINGS

In its simplest form, gratitude journalling is incredibly time-effective, requiring only a few minutes as you list three things, or facts, or people, you are grateful for. The effects, however, are far from insignificant – involving shifting from a lack mindset to an abundance mindset, which not only boosts happiness levels but also makes you more sociable and contributes to long-term permanent change.

Some morning meditators and workout enthusiasts incorporate gratitude into their morning rituals by simply having a moment of gratitude at the end of their daily practice. Keen writers, on the other hand, have been known to take gratitude journalling to a whole new level, writing pages about what makes them feel blessed every morning. What they all agree on is this: a little bit of gratitude can go a long way toward fundamentally changing the way you look at the world.

"When you arise in the morning, think of what a precious privilege it is to be alive - to breathe, to think, to enjoy, to love."
— MARCUS AURELIUS

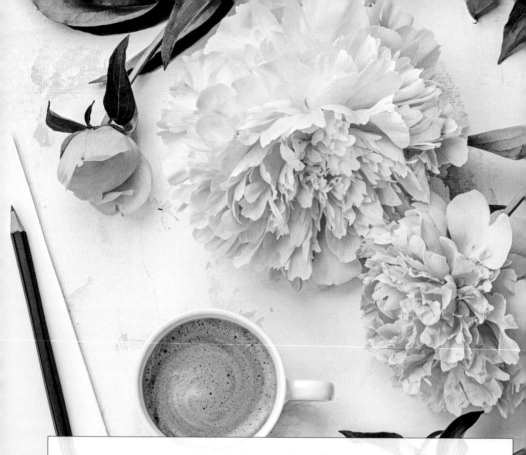

Scarcity vs abundance

Living with a lack-based or scarcity mindset means allowing negative feelings to determine the narrative of your life. It is a fear-based experience of not having enough, focusing on the things you are missing and feel you can't achieve.

A gratitude practice can help you shift to an abundance mindset where challenges are seen as opportunities, you cherish the people and things you already have in life and you adopt a proactive rather than reactive attitude. This in turn makes you more generous and able to genuinely celebrate the successes and happiness of others, as you know that there is an abundance of love and goodness in the world.

WRITING A GRATITUDE JOURNAL

Certain journalling habits might appeal to you more than others, and it is advisable to trust your gut and go where your creative juices take you. But before you find your own personal word flow, try it out, play around with a few exercises, stay open-minded - and see where it takes you.

WHAT IS IT?
Choose a pen you love and a new notebook that inspires you. If the thought of ruining a beautiful book makes you anxious, any old piece of paper will do.

WHERE SHOULD I DO IT?
Give yourself a few minutes as you wake up, perhaps staying in bed to keep warm under the duvet, or wrapping up in a dressing gown and sitting in a favourite armchair. If you find that you thrive on more than a few minutes of writing, moving to a dedicated desk space might be a good idea – perhaps with a mug of warm lemon water (see page 110). If you are able to focus with music in the background, you might like to set the scene every morning with a playlist of your favourite calming tunes or an uplifting soundtrack.

HOW DO I DO IT?
At a minimum, make a simple list of those things for which you are grateful today,

including anything from sunny weather to good health. Discovering genuine gratitude for a few things tends to be more beneficial than a long, exhaustive list – plus, being able to make the list quickly might make you more likely to keep it up.

Remember, the key to success is not in *how* you do it, but *that* you do it. This method of retraining the brain to notice and focus on the good things is a real-life example of how what you focus on will grow.

WHO IS IT FOR?
This will suit those with very limited time, whose mood may need a lift. As little as 2 minutes every morning can be enough.

WHAT ARE THE BENEFITS?
For many people, gratitude journalling increases feelings of happiness and contentedness, and some also notice a boost in productivity, motivation and energy levels.

THE ART OF POSITIVE JOURNALLING

With a mother and a sister who experienced bipolar episodes, an awareness of mental health has always been an important aspect of author Megan C Hayes' life. As she studied for her bachelor's degree in creative writing, she came to realize that putting pen to paper was her way of supporting her own mental health and was central to her wellbeing. This prompted her toward a career of research and teaching in this area. Here she shares her journalling tips and views on the emotional benefits of the habit.

ON WRITING FOR POSITIVITY

"Writing – in a journal or more creatively – can encourage positive emotional intelligence. My book Write Yourself Happy focuses a lot on journalling and also introduces the idea of writing creatively as a path to wellbeing. Journals often risk becoming repositories for all our negative feelings, but when we journal we don't just write ourselves; we become readers of ourselves, and continually re-reading only our gloominess can feel deeply negative.

"Looking to our diverse positive emotions helps to illuminate the intricacies of happiness. Hope springs from bad times, but it is ultimately positive; serenity is a positive emotion that is much quieter than, say, joy. A journal can help us to uncover this nuance."

WHY JOURNAL IN THE MORNING?

"Anything I do in the morning sets the tone for the day. We can use journalling in the morning to refocus ourselves and prioritize the positive emotions we want to feel, such as hope (see opposite). This way we're not just batting back experiences but feel in charge and directed."

TIPS FOR JOURNALLING NOVICES

- "Make it as pleasurable as possible – such as writing while cosy in bed. We are drawn to pleasurable things, so if it feels like a chore you won't keep it up. Focus on the joy of it."

- "Refrain from trying to keep it neat and beautiful. Don't be afraid of making a mess – you don't have to share it on Instagram."

- "Counter self-censorship by writing on loose sheets of paper that you can discard if you wish."

Writing "hope"*

In your journal, write about what hope feels like, looks like, tastes like or smells like using imaginative detail and description. Is hope a seductive shade of silver or a bright and sunny yellow? Does it taste syrupy or zesty? Let any new imagery sit with you for a while, then ask yourself which one feels poignant. This may well form the basis of a more creative piece of writing, such as a poem, and if it does, that's great.

Once you have written about hope in these novel ways, you may like to write about something specific that you are hopeful about in your life. What will you do to meet this goal? Who will help you get there? What personal resources can you call upon, such as your bravery or self-compassion?

*Adapted from an exercise in Write Yourself Happy: The Art of Positive Journalling, by Megan C Hayes

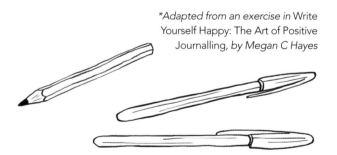

MINI RITUALS FOR THE BRAIN

There is nothing to say that you have to miss out on mental clarity just because you can't seem to get into the writing habit or the family morning schedule is just too tight. Start small with one of these quick and simple ways to get focused, or incorporate them into another type of morning ritual. There is power in the little things.

LIST YOUR VALUES

On a piece of paper or a postcard, list your core values, and then put the list on the inside of your wardrobe. Every morning as you get dressed, read one or more of these values out loud or to yourself. A simple reminder can be enough to put you in the right, truthful frame of mind. If you are more of a visual person, drawing simple symbols that trigger the feelings of these values can work a treat, too.

AFFIRMATION STICKY NOTES

Affirmations (see page 57) are a bit like declarations, but always positive and personal. If you are under a lot of pressure, you might choose to work with an affirmation such as "I am resilient" or "I am calm", while a post-illness affirmation may be "I am strong". You can choose to focus on more than one affirmation at any one time, but make sure that they are specific and relevant to your life and emotional space at that moment – then write them down on sticky notes and position them in places where you know you'll spend time every morning, such as by the bedside table, on the bathroom mirror or where you leave your keys.

MAKE A GRATITUDE LIST

Another list to put up at home, perhaps on the refrigerator, the gratitude list is a simple way to incorporate gratitude into your morning without the journalling or quite as much work. By listing categories such as people, material items and skills, you can pick just one to focus on as you get breakfast or coffee every morning. One day you might acknowledge a long-standing friendship; another day it might be your health. Insignificant though it may seem, this quick exercise still trains your brain to focus on what you have and what is possible, instead of spiralling into stress and worry.

STRIKE A POWER POSE

Stand proudly with your feet firmly on the ground with your legs wider than your hips, back straight, chest out and chin up. Raise your arms up in a V shape above your head, or pull back your shoulders and open your arms out wide to the sides, as if about to embrace someone. Take a deep breath. Smile. Say an affirmation out loud if you have one. Try to remember this feeling as and when you need it throughout your day.

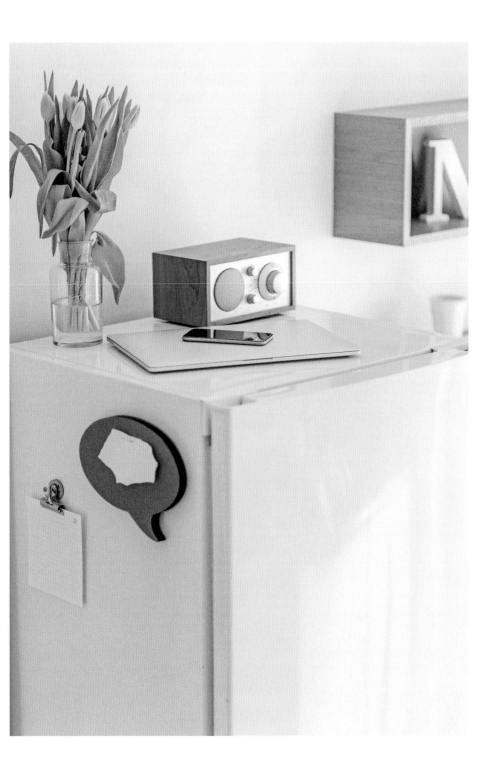

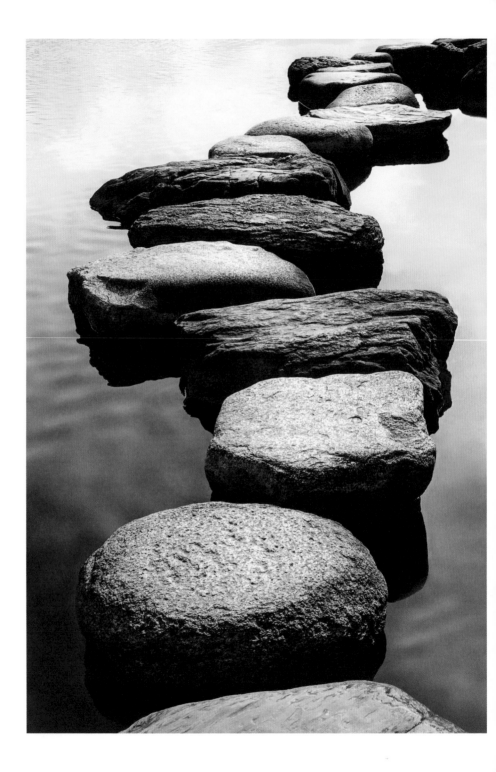

SET A GOAL –
AND MEAN IT

Some say that the reason gratitude journalling is so effective is the fact that it tugs at the heartstrings - it really means something to us. That is why goal setting, if you want to get maximum benefit from it, should do the very same.

Some might say that goal setting is a form of escapism, that the journey is overlooked as you reach for a distant future. On the contrary, daily victory on a meaningful path is a good place to be.

GOALS FOR YOU

- Where best to start? Ideally, way ahead in the future – maybe ten years from now.

- What do you want it to look like? This is big work, no doubt about it. Think family, career, fitness, societal contribution and life purpose – all the things that might be important to you, the things you are deeply passionate about.

- Once you know where you're headed, trace your steps back via a series of small goals: where will you need to be in two years' time to reach that goal? Where does that leave your six-monthly and then your weekly goals?

- As you achieve these part-goals – one by one, day by day, week by week, year by year – they take you closer to the next one, and to that vision of yours.

BE SMART

Anyone who has ever worked in project management will know that a goal must always be SMART: Specific, Measurable, Attainable, Realistic and Timely. And behind each goal is a series of tasks – steps for you to take and tick off on a daily basis in order to reach your goal. If your goal is really SMART and you are truly motivated to reach it, there is very little to suggest that you will fail.

But more than just getting you from A to B, good goal setting saves you a lot of time. You can keep very busy without getting very far, but once you weed out the distraction work from the crucial tasks, you can prioritize better and keep your focus clear. Review your tasks daily, always in line with your big-picture goals.

The brain thrives on victory – and here is the perfect opportunity to help it flourish. Achieving every small goal is a victory in itself, complete with a confidence boost and a top-up in motivation.

PICTURE THIS

When we say goals should tug at the heartstrings, what do we mean? What stops you from abandoning a goal is that gnawing feeling in your gut that tells you that this is too important to let go of. The technique of visualization is used for this purpose: to help you see, feel and connect with your goal; to know that it matters; and to feel that it's possible to reach it.

Visualization is commonly used in sports and by successful entrepreneurs to provide a clearer focus and boost confidence. It has also proved useful for helping stroke patients who have suffered tissue death in a limb; imagining themselves moving that limb actually reduces tissue loss in the surrounding area. This is because neurons in our brain don't always differentiate between visualized imagery and real-life action – so when you imagine doing something, the part of your brain that would be activated when actually doing it is stimulated. If you keep visualizing something happening, your brain will think it possible.

In addition to its value to neuroscience, visualization boosts your motivation and triggers your creative subconscious. If gratitude journalling brings your attention to what's good in life, a clearly visualized goal can alert you to relevant opportunities you don't want to miss.

Visualization techniques to try out

1. For the simplest kind of visualization practice, adopt a comfortable, seated position, close your eyes and picture in great detail your goal as if it had already been achieved. This is best done first thing in the morning when you are at your most relaxed.

2. Using image manipulation software, you can create pictures of yourself in your dream scenarios, be it wearing the graduation cap of your university of choice or standing outside your perfect home in your chosen location. Create one for every aspect of your life and look at them every morning.

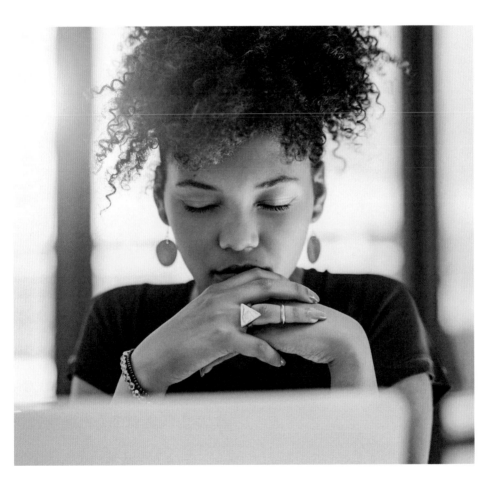

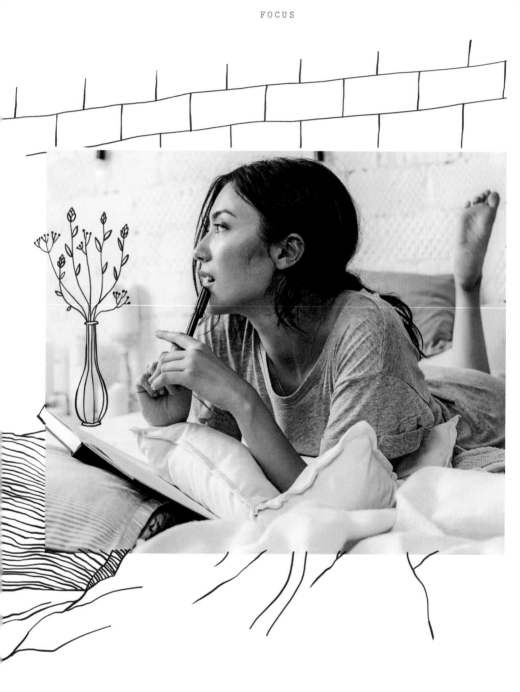

TIPS AND RESOURCES FOR A RITUAL OF CLARITY AND FOCUS

If you know you want to try out some journalling or goal setting but you're not sure where to start, play around with one or more of the following exercises to see what sticks.

- Think of a positive experience from the previous day, when you felt empowered, happy or calm. Describe what happened and how you felt.

- Clarify your intentions. What do you want to feel like, and how do you want to be? Intentions are typically more far-reaching and values-based than daily or even weekly goals are, but reminding yourself of the values you intend to embody is a huge step toward reaching those goals.

- Look at the things you are grateful for then consider what your life would be like without them. This can help stop you taking for granted the positive aspects of your life.

- Get creative. Draw your gratitude instead of writing it. Perhaps sing it or dance it – make sure you really feel and embody it.

- Type out your goals on cards. Read these every morning, then visualize each goal being reached.

- Picture yourself on the day you retire: imagine what you look like, where you live and how you spend your time. Consider what this "future you" would think of where

you are at today – your goals, fears and dreams. How can this "future you" help guide the present you toward what really matters? What will you be grateful for on the eve of your retirement?

IF YOU ONLY DO ONE THING...
When you wake up in the morning, sit for 2 minutes on the edge of the bed, close your eyes and think of one thing you are grateful for. Take that gratitude with you into your day.

What you need

Journalling, planning and goal setting are low-maintenance and low-cost practices. A pen and piece of paper go a long way; even a notebook won't set you back much. Add a little bit of motivation and discipline, and you're all set.

FOCUS – SUGGESTED RITUALS

Let a pen and your dreams lead the way

Adapt the ritual suggestions below to suit what you're looking for, be it gratitude, productivity or a clear mind. Journalling and visualization can be done anywhere, so all you need to do is decide how much time you can commit to your practice, and then find your groove.

RITUAL FOR THE TIME-POOR

– Keep a notepad by your bedside and, when you wake up, take a moment to think about and jot down three things you are grateful for (see page 91).

– Take that gratitude with you as you get dressed and make breakfast, perhaps adding some nut butter or fresh berries to a chia pudding prepared the night before (see page 114).

– After you brush your teeth, say an affirmation (see page 57) in front of the bathroom mirror to get you in the right headspace for the day ahead.

– If you have a presentation or important meeting ahead of you, visualize yourself in action while on your way into work, and picture what the ideal situation looks like.

RITUAL FOR THE TIME-RICH

– Get comfortable and empty your mind into your favourite notebook. You could look to Julia Cameron's morning pages for inspiration (see page 89).

– Spend a few minutes visualizing a best-case scenario for the day ahead, be it a successful presentation, a calm and focused day of work or a way of dealing with a colleague or loved one you've been thinking about (see page 100).

– Have a wash or a shower and bring yourself out of that cosy morning mindset with a face rinse, eye wash, and ear massage (see page 131).

– Enjoy a breakfast of your choice (for inspiration, see page 114).

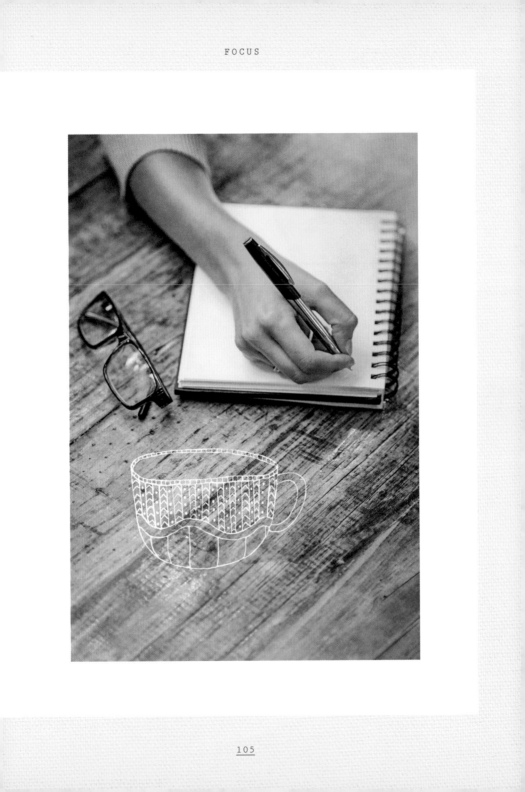

"One cannot think
well, love well,
sleep well, if one
has not dined well."
— VIRGINIA WOOLF

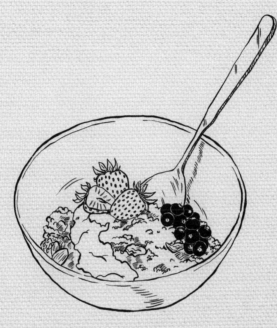

CHAPTER 5

NOURISH

Rituals for the gut

BREAKING THE FAST

I think rooibos might be my favourite tea colour: I love to see the warm, rich, fiery-brown whirls of nutty flavour moving through the water as the tea brews. I was never a big tea drinker, but that friend who gave me a glass teapot knew about the mindful act of watching tea darken.

Add the peace and quiet of a home still asleep, a village where only the rooster is starting to wake up, or a city in stillness, waiting to stir. Combining that potent calm with the soft movement of brewing tea will help you understand why early risers tend to prefer tea over coffee.

I grew up with the notion that breakfast is the most important meal of the day, and on most mornings I was barely awake for 15 minutes before I was at the kitchen table with a bowl of muesli. Breakfast was a thing to get through, a step on the necessary journey from getting out of bed to walking out the door. I never really minded it but can't say I ever paid much attention to it either.

Now that I'm raising two kids on porridge with apple and seeds, all too often hurrying them to keep moving in case we run late, I'm thinking more about what we put into our bodies. Maybe I hadn't thought enough about what a rushed meal does to metabolism, not to mention cortisol levels, and how nagging and prodding set the tone for the day. Never once did I think that breaking the fast a little later in the morning would even be an option, let alone watching tea darken in all its glory.

For fellow parents of young children and others struggling to get out the door on time, a good place to start might be to become aware of what breakfast feels like – and then simply try to make it feel good.

"Let food be thy medicine
and medicine be thy food."
— HIPPOCRATES

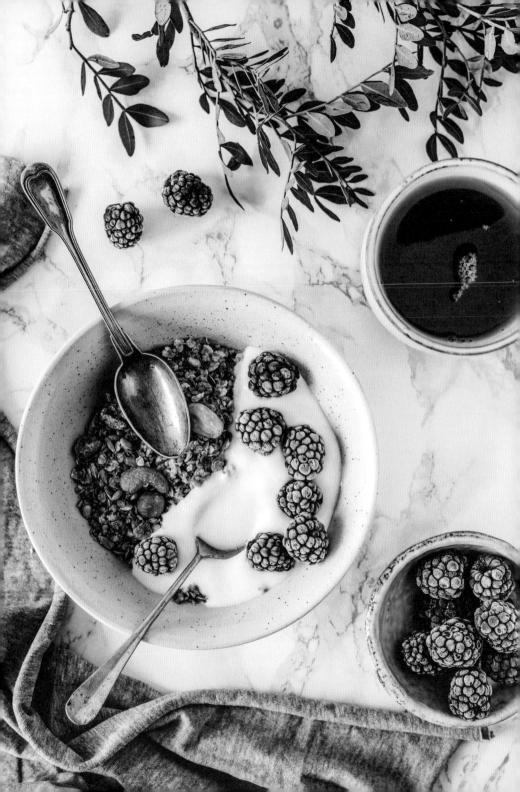

WHEN LIFE GIVES YOU LEMONS, BOIL THE KETTLE

Yogis, journallers, meditators - many morning ritual enthusiasts have one thing in common: they start every morning with a glass of warm water with lemon. Countless nutritionists are humming to the same tune.

One of the most important things when you wake up in the morning is hydration. We are dehydrated because we haven't been drinking for hours and have been sweating in our sleep. When we drink, we rehydrate the body's cells and kickstart our metabolism, telling our body that we're ready for a new day.

A drink of water reduces your heart rate and increases blood flow to the brain, thereby boosting the flow of oxygen in the body and the production of red blood cells. Add lemon to the mix and you've got yourself a true morning tonic, not just refreshing in flavour but renewing and healing in countless ways.

If you're just getting used to rising early, lemon water alone can function as an effective mini ritual. The preparation of your lemon drink will quickly become second nature, and the fact that you are starting out the same way every day, with an act of self-care, will have a calming effect and invite you to enjoy a few mindful minutes.

Why add lemon to your morning tipple?

1. Lemons are rich in vitamin C, which boosts your immune system, has an anti-inflammatory effect and helps the body absorb iron from other foods.

2. Lemons, counterintuitively, have an alkaline effect on the body, helping to balance pH levels.

3. Lemons have a diuretic effect and help the body to flush out toxins.

How to drink it

Squeeze the juice of half a lemon into a glass.

Fill half the glass with boiling water, then top it up with cold tap water. Alternatively, heat the water in a pan to just above lukewarm and fill up the glass.

Drink - and enjoy.

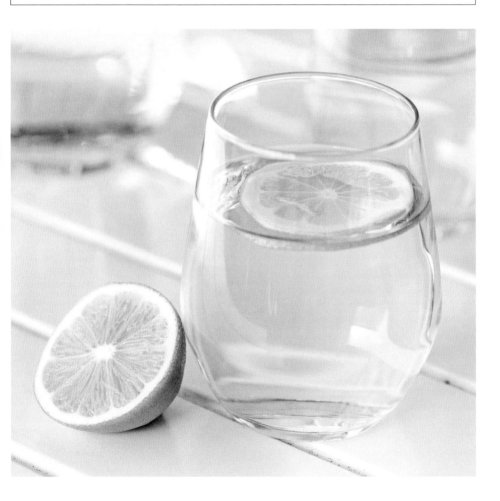

SUPERFOOD INSPIRATION

What do you put into your body? Does it serve you well? What might you be missing out on? Here are some superfoods (food with a nutritional composition that has health benefits or disease-fighting properties) that would make good additions to your morning nourishment.

AVOCADO
Joke all you want about the hipster avocado habit stopping young people from getting on the property ladder, but there's a reason why everyone loves them – and it's not just because they taste great. Rich in fibre and monounsaturated fats, avocados are good for your heart, make you feel full for longer and contribute a long list of important vitamins, including many of the B complex that are otherwise difficult to get. Add magnesium, zinc and all sorts of other goodness and you'll see why this belongs on the superfood list.

GINGER
Gorgeous ginger provides plenty of antioxidants and anti-inflammatory properties (helping to reduce inflammation in the body, which sometimes develops in response to injury or as part of other healing processes), it also gives a welcome kick to smoothies and hot drinks. Some people find that ginger helps settle nausea and heartburn, and it's also said to balance the gut and help with everything from diarrhea to constipation.

KALE
Kale contains heaps of vitamins as well as calcium, potassium and iron, all in addition to ultra-healthy fibre. It's truly a superfood for the heart as well as the digestive system.

TURMERIC
Everyone's talking about turmeric – and for good reason. For a long time, it has played a big role in Ayurvedic medicine, an ancient tradition of medicine with its roots in the Indian subcontinent. Amazing for reducing joint pain – thanks to its anti-inflammatory properties – and restoring cartilage, turmeric is best enjoyed along with black pepper to improve uptake.

CHILLI
Not everyone is open to the idea of starting the day with chilli, but if you are, a smoothie with a kick might be just the thing for you. Chillies are rich in capsaicin, which boosts endorphin levels and works as a natural painkiller. Like many of the other superfoods, chilli has anti-inflammatory benefits.

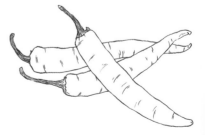

Add, don't restrict

Research on the psychological consequences of food restriction (which can involve, for example, eliminating entire food groups or avoiding certain nutritional forms) shows that it rarely has the desired effects and can contribute to eating disorders. Stop thinking about how you want to limit what you eat and focus instead on the goodness you want to try to add to your diet. The long-term benefits are often much greater, as is the chance that you'll create lasting habits.

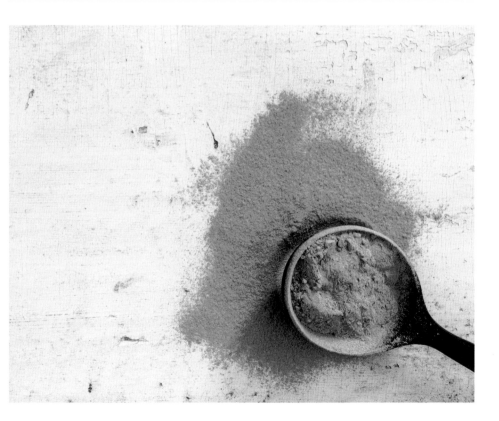

EVERYDAY BREAKFAST

For a quick breakfast that sets you up well for the day, try one of these simple but nurturing ideas.

CREAMY GREEN SMOOTHIE

Start your day with a blend of folate, fibre, vitamin C, iron and much more with this green smoothie that has all the goodness of avocado and spinach. For a flavour-and-endorphin boost, add a little bit of chilli and ginger.

Serves 2

1 avocado, peeled and stoned
juice of 1 lime
30g (1¼oz) spinach
2 celery sticks
25g (1oz) parsley
1 teaspoon green powder such as spirulina, wheatgrass or chlorella
Salt and pepper
2cm (¾in) piece of peeled fresh root ginger (optional)
half a deseeded red chilli (optional)

Place all the ingredients in a food processor or blender with enough water to cover. Process until smooth. Season to taste and blend again. Pour into two glasses and serve.

CHIA PUDDING

Used by the Aztecs for centuries, chia seeds are rich in omega-3 fatty acids, fibre and protein as well as a number of minerals. They are known for their anti-inflammatory properties and benefits for the heart.

Serves 2

PUDDING BASE
6 tablespoons chia seeds
450ml (15fl oz) milk of your choice
local honey, to taste (optional)

TOPPINGS (OPTIONAL)
nut butter; cinnamon; fresh fruit or berries

The night before, combine the chia seeds and milk, or put in a jar and shake. Leave to set overnight. In the morning, add your toppings.

For a super boost

Add goji berries to your chia pudding or overnight oats. They are rich in everything from antioxidants to minerals, and are a super source of vitamin C.

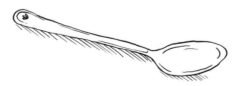

OTHER BREAKFAST IDEAS

Overnight oats: Mix 45g (1½oz) oats with 1 tablespoon chia seeds and 125ml (4fl oz) of your milk of choice (see box, right). Refrigerate overnight. In the morning, add berries, a sliced banana, a pinch of cinnamon or a big spoonful of peanut butter.

Shakes and smoothies: These can be made from any vegetables and fruit you have. For example, put as a base a handful of spinach or kale, plus some fresh parsley and an apple, in a blender. Squeeze in some fresh lime juice, and grate in some ginger. Just cover with almond milk or water, then blend. If you like a little bit of sweetness, you could try a banana and peanut butter base instead of the greens.

Eggs, nuts and half a grapefruit: Having boiled eggs ready in the fridge is useful for

mornings when time is short. Nuts provide endless benefits thanks to plenty of fibre, healthy fats, vitamins and minerals, and are said to be at their most beneficial if eaten in the morning. Half a grapefruit boasts more than a third of your daily recommended vitamin C.

Choosing milk

Cashew milk is deliciously creamy, while oat milk is gentler on the environment, especially if you can find a brand that's produced near you.

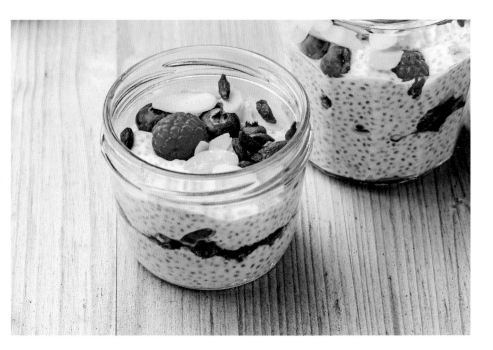

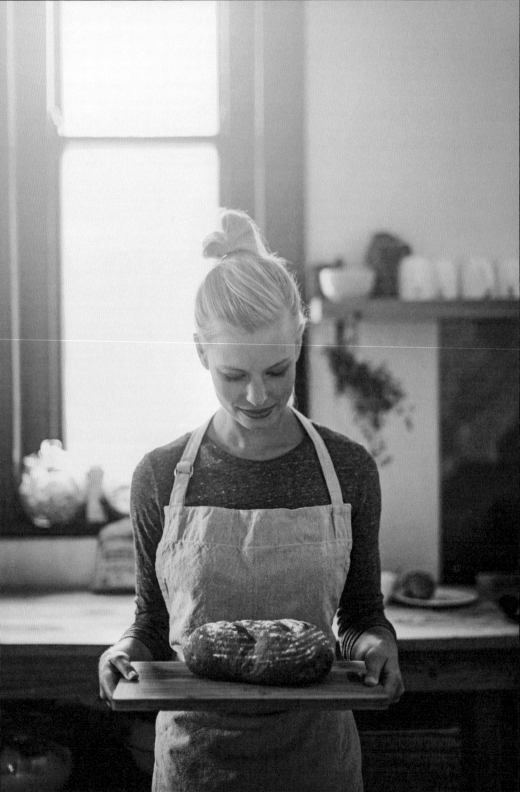

WHOLESOME WEEKEND RITUALS

―――――――――

A friend of mine has the loveliest ritual: every Saturday morning, she meets her best friends for brunch. They are all busy career women, so they don't get to catch up during the week. This brunch date is a commitment to friendship and gorgeous food. If rituals are about identity, presence and committing to what matters most to you, this ticks all the boxes. Not everyone can afford brunch in a restaurant every Saturday, but making time for getting together with friends, enjoying quality time with a favourite weekend newspaper or indulging in some baking are surely self-care rituals we can all get behind.

SUNFLOWER SEED AND RYE BREAD
If you want a change from chia pudding and overnight oats (see pages 114 and 115), why not do some baking, enjoying the smell of freshly baked bread filling your home?

Makes 1 loaf

200g (7oz) plain flour
200g (7oz) wholemeal spelt flour
100g (3½oz) rye flour
2 teaspoons baking powder
1 teaspoon salt
75g (3oz) sunflower seeds, plus extra to sprinkle
500g (1lb) natural yogurt
milk, to glaze

Preheat the oven to 220°C/425°F/Gas Mark 7. Grease a 1.25kg (2½lb) loaf tin.

Mix together the flours, baking powder, salt and sunflower seeds in a bowl. Stir in the yogurt and mix to a fairly soft dough.

Shape the dough into a log on a floured surface, then drop into the prepared tin. Brush with a little milk and sprinkle with the remaining sunflower seeds.

Bake for 20 minutes. Reduce the oven temperature to 160°C/325°F/Gas Mark 3, and bake for a further 30 minutes. The bread is done when the base sounds hollow when tapped, so, if necessary, return to the oven for a little longer. Transfer to a wire rack to cool.

A NUTRITIONIST ON GUT-FRIENDLY MORNINGS

Jenny Tschiesche is an author, nutritionist, recipe developer and speaker. Here, she advises on what to (or not to) eat and drink to wake up your body and metabolism, for the best possible start and sustained energy throughout the day.

SETTING THE TONE FOR THE DAY
"The first thing we eat sets the tone for the rest of the day. If we get up and have something sugary, something based on refined carbs, it's going to raise the level of glucose in the body. We'll react by producing insulin to bring it down – but we might overcompensate and end up with plummeting blood sugar, and then we turn to sugar and caffeine to get that boost. It gets us into a trap that affects our performance whatever we do."

ON WAKING UP THE BODY
"A lot of people start their day with coffee to get that hit, but we need water to hydrate in the morning. If you have something like lemon water or even cucumber water, it can have a cleansing effect while waking up the body after hours of sleep. Moreover, coffee is similar

to sugar in that it's a stimulant, and having too many stimulants sets you off on this roller coaster of highs and lows – it's not good!"

WHAT TO EAT IN THE MORNING
"Breakfast doesn't need to take place early in the morning, and I understand that not everyone wants a big bowl of porridge first thing – but looking at overall health and metabolism, everyone needs a decent amount of protein and fibre. Kefir (a fermented milk drink) is a favourite of mine; it's high in protein but also has probiotic bacteria that is great for gut health. Eggs are great too, as is anything with flax seeds, chia seeds or oats, and seeds and nuts."

JENNY'S BREAKFAST TIPS
Eggs in every way: "Keep them in the refrigerator, hard-boiled or soft-boiled, and enjoy for breakfast along with any leftover veg you may have from the night before."

Plantain or under-ripe banana omelette: "Resistant starches in plantains and under-ripe bananas are great prebiotics (compounds that boost the growth and activity of beneficial bacteria), which fuel probiotics (microorganisms that help restore and improve the gut flora)."

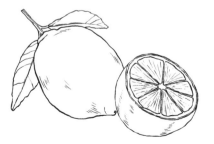

Grate-and-infuse drink: *"For a fresh start to your day, you can't go far wrong with ginger, lemon or turmeric 'tea'. To prepare in advance, grate some fresh ginger, lemon peel or fresh turmeric using the coarse setting on your grater. Store the gratings, individually or mixed together, in the freezer (you can use the compartments of an ice cube tray for this). In the morning, simply place some gratings in a mug, or put them in a tea infuser, and add warm water. A twist of black pepper will give your tea a little extra zing (and is a perfect pairing for turmeric, as it helps absorption)."*

A fruitful tip

As a rule of thumb, fruit is higher in sugar the closer it grows to the equator, so choose Nordic berries over fruit from near the equator if you can.

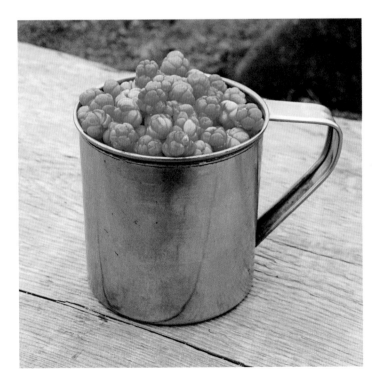

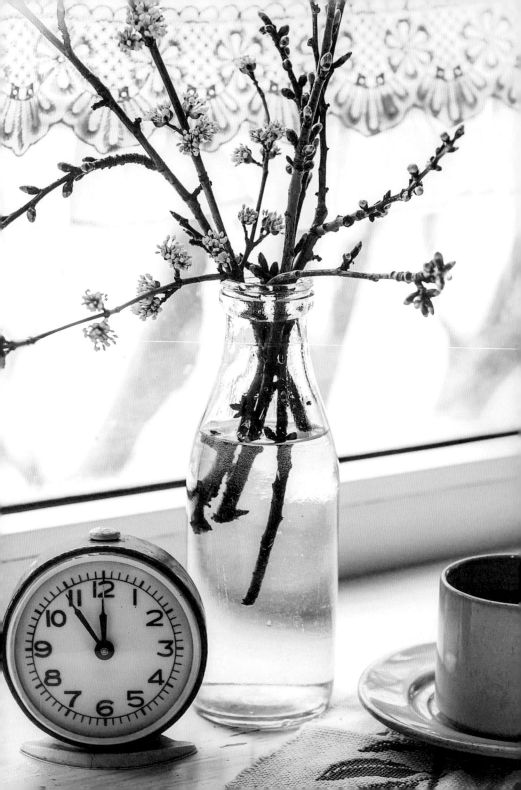

A WORD ON INTERMITTENT FASTING

Breakfast is the first thing we eat when we break the fast of sleep, but there's nothing to say that you have to eat breakfast in the morning. In fact, more and more people are choosing not to, but is fasting just a fad or should we be paying attention? Nutritionist Jenny Tschiesche (see page 118) thinks we should, but with a good sprinkling of patience and self-awareness.

One of the most popular forms of intermittent fasting is the 16:8 approach, which means that in every 24 hours you fast for 16 hours straight and eat for 8. The benefits include optimized metabolism as you give the gut a proper chance to do its thing and learn how to cope without food.

That said, most of us have been socialized to start out with a bowl of porridge or something similar first thing in the morning and to end with a big meal at night, or perhaps even an early evening dinner followed by a late snack before we go to bed. In the spirit of realism and self-kindness, take an honest look at how you eat, when you eat, and why. Do you need to have your biggest meal of the day in the evening, when your body is meant to start to slow down, or could you have it for lunch? If your breakfast routine is dictated by your commute and work hours, could you perhaps drop that late-night snack and give your gut a break that way?

Forget cutting calories and going hungry; this isn't about banning meals and food groups. But by becoming conscious of your eating habits, you might be able to cut the amazing machine that is your body some well-deserved slack, and feel all the better for it.

"Our bodies are our gardens, to which our wills are gardeners."
— WILLIAM SHAKESPEARE

NUTRITION TIPS

*It's not just about what you eat - but also when you eat it,
how you eat it, and in what context. Here are some tips
on how to make the most of that breakfast ritual.*

DID YOU KNOW?

- Research suggests that our breakfast choices influence our sleep. For a good night's rest, avoid diets that are high in saturated fats and sugar, and increase your fibre intake. Also, follow nutritionist Jenny Tschiesche's tips (see page 118) to avoid a blood sugar roller coaster.

- If you eat quickly, your body doesn't produce enough enzymes and hydrochloric acid to break down the food sufficiently as it passes through the gut.

- Studies have shown that, if we rush a meal and don't eat mindfully, the body doesn't always prioritize digestion. If our mind is stressing about something, the body will prioritize dealing with the stress over digestion, leading to fermentation of food in the gut and a build-up of gas.

IF YOU EXERCISE...

Exercising on an empty stomach is fine if you can't face eating first thing or you're simply a fan of fasted training, but always remember to drink before your workout. Post-exercise, help the body to recover with a combination of carbohydrates and protein. Porridge with berries and a generous spoonful of nut butter is a great option.

DOS AND DON'TS

- Don't waste money on bottled super-juices and expensive energy bars that you could just as easily make yourself in a big batch at home. Healthy morning nutrition doesn't have to cost a fortune, nor does it need to depend on a booming multi-trillion-dollar wellness industry.

- Do listen to your body. If you need an early breakfast, have an early breakfast. If porridge makes you bloated, eat something else. Being aware of how you start your day doesn't mean doing what others tell you to do or banning food groups – but it can help you tell the difference between habits created by a mind that's playing tricks on you and your body's true signals.

IF YOU ONLY DO ONE THING...
Drink a big glass of water, with or without lemon, as soon as you wake up. Few things will work as they should if you are dehydrated and therefore short on many of the salts that the body needs.

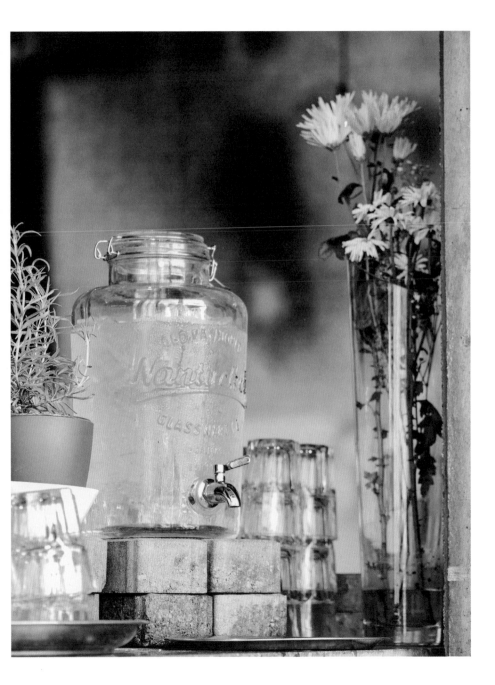

NOURISH – SUGGESTED RITUALS
Rituals for minding the machine that is your body

From your energy levels to your ability to think clearly, so much of your wellbeing is directly linked to nourishment and what you eat. Whatever tips and tricks you use to wake up the body and focus the mind, you can incorporate parts of these suggested rituals to get a holistically sound start to your day.

RITUAL FOR THE TIME-POOR

– As you get ready, before brushing your teeth, do some oil pulling (see page 132) to detoxify and contribute to better breath all day.

– Try to make time for having breakfast mindfully in order to allow the body to do its job properly (read more on page 118) – just make sure to prepare a chia pudding or some overnight oats (see pages 114 and 115) the night before, and all it requires is a few minutes of being fully present at the breakfast table.

– Hold off on the coffee until you start work (see page 118).

– Now that your body has been fed and nourished, settle into a mindfulness of breathing meditation (see page 47) on the bus or train into work, or at your desk before you start work.

RITUAL FOR THE TIME-RICH

– Rise early, before everyone else in the house if you can.

– Prepare a grate-and-infuse drink (see page 119) with warm water, then sit down in a cosy corner or go outside to catch the first birdsong.

– Take a moment to clarify your intentions (see page 57) – what you want to feel like and how you want to be as you face your day.

– Put on your favourite radio station or podcast and prepare some scrambled eggs or an omelette (see page 118).

– Add some cacao butter to your coffee – it's known to slow down the uptake of caffeine and provide the body with a slow-release form of energy.

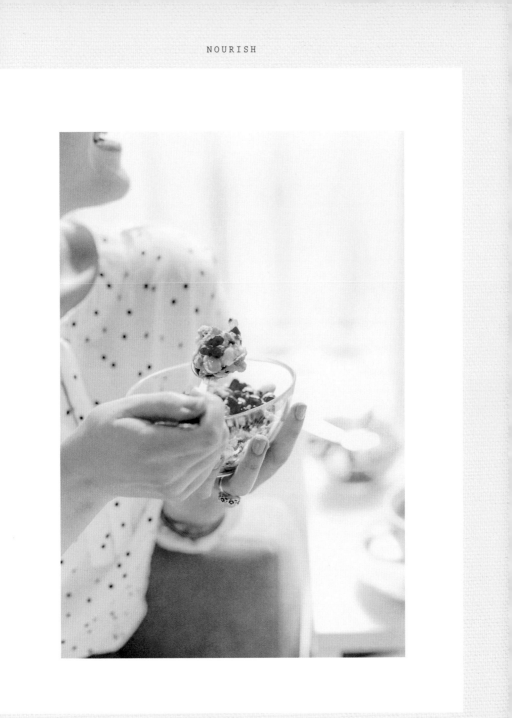

"Clean out your ears,
don't listen for what
you already know."

— RUMI

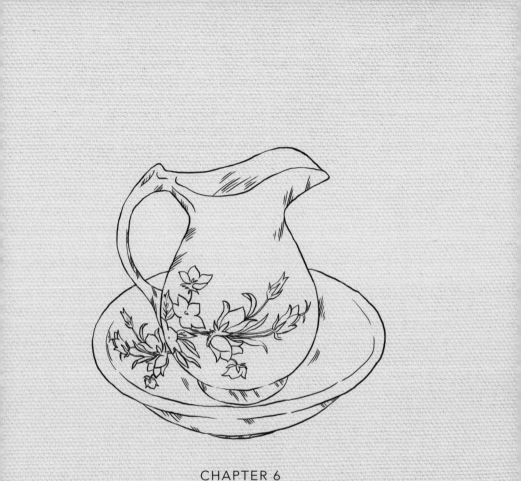

CHAPTER 6

CLEANSE

Washing, oiling
and rehydrating

SELF-CARE ACCORDING TO AYURVEDA

In Ayurveda, a cleansing ritual is seen as a way to get a head start by aligning the body with nature's rhythms and the doshas *(biological energies in the human body and mind, derived from the five elements) first thing every morning.*

The Sanskrit word *ayurveda* means knowledge of life and longevity, and the key to a good life and good health, according to this philosophy, is to live in tune with nature's cycles. This includes rising and setting with the sun and trying to balance the three *doshas* – *vata*, *pitta* and *kapha* – so they are as close to your natural *dosha* state as possible. Put simply, the thinking is that our unique combination of the *doshas* defines our personality, and that external factors such as stress and particular diets can throw us off balance.

RISE WITH *VATA*

In Ayurvedic thought, the hours before dawn are dominated by a vibrant *vata* energy, making it easier to rise at this time. The peace and quiet of pre-dawn morning time also makes it conducive to meditation (see page 41) and *pranayama* (see page 34), whereas waking after dawn, when a heavy *kapha* energy dominates, makes you feel sluggish. Try rising 20 minutes or so before dawn for some inward contemplation and breathing before starting your cleansing ritual.

INCORPORATING AYURVEDA IN YOUR MORNING RITUAL

A dedicated Ayurvedic morning ritual takes time – often hours – as well as study and training. Not only do you need to get to know your own natural *dosha* state better (see box opposite) in order to design a ritual that really benefits you, but the ritual is also likely to include an extended series of activities in addition to a full body cleanse, covering everything from meditation and movement to nourishment.

A different approach is to choose freely from the many indulgent aspects of Ayurvedic cleansing to find a morning ritual that simply feels great. We will explore a number of these throughout this chapter. Read on, and try the ones that resonate most strongly with you.

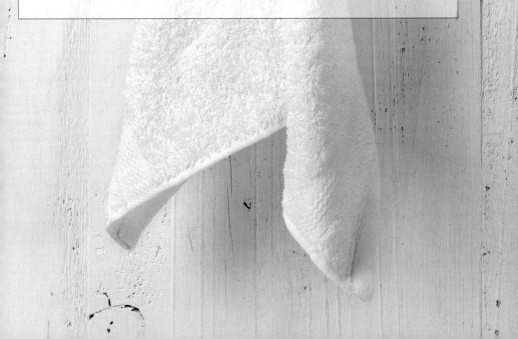

The three *doshas*

1. *Vata:* The energy of movement, characterized by the mobile nature of the elements of space and air.

2. *Pitta:* The energy of digestion and metabolism, derived from the transformative nature of the elements of fire and water.

3. *Kapha:* The energy of building, binding and lubrication, like a glue for smooth functioning of the entire body, derived from the elements of water and earth.

Discover your *dosha* constitution by taking this online quiz: www.ayurvedichealthcenter.com/determine-your-dosha.

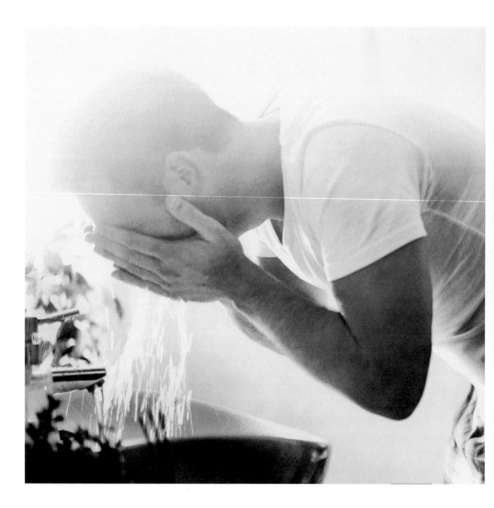

REVIVING SKIN, EARS AND EYES

*Wash the night away the Ayurvedic way. A gentle
morning cleanse, incorporating a splash of water
across your face, circular movements massaging your
temples and a touch of lavender oil behind your ears,
can be the most nourishing version of self-care.*

FACE RINSE

Dry air, old pillows, sweat and dust – we
often talk about beauty sleep, but the truth
is that our skin puts up with a lot at night.
Ayurveda describes face rinsing as a way to
wash away *pitta* energy and prepare the skin
for the demands of the day ahead. The
recommended treatment is to splash the face
with cold water seven times (once for each of
the body's chakras, or energy centres). Taking
a sip of water, swishing it around and spitting it
out is also recommended as part of the rinse,
since the entire body wakes up dehydrated.

EAR MASSAGE

If you suffer from a stiff neck or jaw, try this
quick yet surprisingly pleasant and relaxing
ear massage. Using your thumb and index
finger, rub the rim of each ear, starting at the
top and working your way down. Take a few
drops of sesame oil and rub it just outside
the opening of the ear canal. This practice,
known as *Karna Puran*, or *Karna Purana*, is
used in Ayurveda to treat ailments resulting
from increased *vata* energy. You can also
rub a few drops of sesame oil just inside your
nostrils to benefit your sinuses and your mind.

EYE WASH

The eyes are the seat of the *pitta dosha*,
or the seat of fire – and so *pitta* imbalance
is to blame for the majority of eye problems.
Simply splashing your open eyes with water
is thought to help balance the *doshas*.
Particularly puffy eyes can be remedied with
cotton pads soaked in fennel tea or aloe vera
– or the old trick of slices of cool cucumber
can work a treat. If it feels good, gently
massage your eyelids. Follow the eye wash
and massage with an eye workout: move your
eyes from side to side and up and down, and
then roll them both ways. End by squeezing
your eyes shut and quickly opening them
seven times.

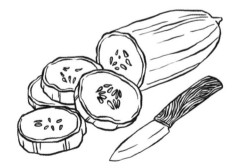

BOOSTING ORAL HEALTH

The two Ayurvedic practices of oil pulling and tongue scraping are very simple to perform and yet highly effective ways of looking after the health of your mouth and, therefore, also your general health. Build them into your morning ritual and you won't regret it.

OIL PULLING

The benefits of oil pulling are many and its devotees incredibly enthusiastic. A promise of reduced gum disease and inflammation, less dryness in the mouth and improved breath (not to mention clearer skin all over the body, thanks to toxins being washed away before they are absorbed by the skin) should be enough to get plenty of people curious. Add everything from a detoxifying effect and increased mental clarity to reduced tiredness, anti-inflammatory benefits and improved dental health – as well as its key purpose of daily detoxification – and it's a wonder that we're not all getting in on the act.

Oil pulling works best on an empty stomach, making it a perfect morning ritual activity. The technique couldn't be easier: just take a teaspoon of coconut or sesame oil (you may need to gently warm the coconut oil first for it to become liquid) and swish it around your mouth for no less than 3 minutes. Take care not to swallow it as the purpose is to pull toxins out of the body. Then spit it out, rinse with warm water and move on to tongue scraping. If you have time, a gentle gum massage using oil and small, counterclockwise motions is great for oral health, too.

TONGUE SCRAPING

From poor oral health and sense of taste to a build-up of damaging *ama* (toxins in the form of undigested food products, which Ayurvedic practitioners believe linger in our bodies), there are many reasons why tongue scraping deserves our attention. You can buy a tongue scraper in large pharmacies or online, or simply opt for a stainless-steel spoon. Scrape down the entire tongue, from as far back as possible to the front, using 7 or 14 strokes, once or twice for each of the seven chakras.

For the best results, you need to scrape every time you eat, but scraping in the morning alone can still make a world of difference, in addition to sorting out that white-coated appearance on the tongue. Twice-daily scraping has been shown to reduce the amount of decay-inducing bacteria in the mouth and prevent both cavities and gum disease.

The great toothpaste debate

To use or not to use fluoride - that is the question. Ayurvedic practitioners recommend you employ a natural toothpaste free from fluoride and also free from sodium lauryl sulphate. This chemical, known simply as SLS, is used in all sorts of cosmetics and cleansing products and is believed by some to aggravate and trigger sensitive-skin conditions, such as eczema and psoriasis. Instead, choose a toothpaste incorporating herbs, such as neem or liquorice.

The reason that some holistic dentists, Ayurvedic practitioners and others are advising not to brush with a toothpaste containing fluoride is that fears have grown in recent years around its potentially neurotoxic nature (it is thought to contain toxins that are poisonous or destructive to nerve tissue). This is, however, still controversial. Most dentists and dental associations argue that fluoride is crucial for, among other things, helping young teeth develop strong, healthy enamel, and it also aids remineralization, the natural protection against destructive bacteria.

"To keep the body in good health is a duty, otherwise we shall not be able to keep our mind strong and clear."
— BUDDHA

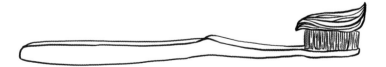

Nourishing oils for your luxury bath

Lavender: for relaxation and reduced stress

Eucalyptus: for renewal and refreshment

Patchouli: for nourishment and harmony

A DAILY FULL-BODY CLEANSE

Most of us start the day with a full-body cleanse in the form of a shower - but some make it count more than others, even opting for a proper, restorative soak or a nourishing oil treatment.

BRACING COLD SHOWERS

The idea of a freezing cold shower might sound extreme, but it has proven benefits, not to mention the fact that it certainly does the job of waking you up. Popularized by Wim Hof, the holder of the world record for the longest ice bath, regular ice-cold showers are said to strengthen your immune system, increase levels of the neurotransmitter dopamine and possibly boost productivity. According to Ayurveda, different *dosha* states (see page 129) benefit from showers of different temperatures, but it's hard to ignore the huge number of people who testify that a cold shower or dip in a wintry sea helps them beat a bad bout of anxiety and depression.

RESTORATIVE BATHS

Soaking in a bath every morning requires more time than a shower, but one complete with essential oils (see box, left) and a body scan meditation (see page 42) can be a wonderful way to start the day when you have enough time and perhaps are yearning for a warming, remedial morning soak. Promoting a moment of mindfulness, baths can be great stress relievers and can also work wonders on aching muscles; some people even suggest they help lower blood sugar levels.

FULL-BODY OIL TREATMENT

Oiling your body can be both relaxing and invigorating. It's also great for tired, dry skin and helps add a protective barrier against toxins. Massaging the skin gets the blood circulation going, so you'll warm up nicely and wake up the body in a wonderfully gentle way – particularly enjoyable if you're just out of a Wim Hof-inspired shower, or if you wake up feeling cold with no time for a full bath ritual.

Warmed organic jojoba or almond oil makes a lovely treatment, perhaps with a drop of an essential oil of your choice mixed in. Start working your way up from your feet with gentle pressure, and pay particular attention to the joints. When you're done, if you can, take 10 minutes to sit still and focus on the sensations in your body. A moment of gratitude may well come naturally.

Remember: anything that you put on your skin will be assimilated by it, so perfumed products and anything containing parabens (widely used preservatives suggested by some to be carcinogenic) and SLS (see page 133) may be best avoided. An extensive range of organic and Ayurvedic soaps and nourishing oils are available.

SMOKE CLEANSING

Smoke cleansing is inspired by ancient practices of burning dried herbs and plants to create a smoke that clears and cleanses a space. Many different herbs can be used, depending on tradition and preference.

WHY DO IT?

Smoke cleansing brings an ethereal ambience similar to when you burn incense, but with added proven benefits for air quality. Notably, the smoke produced is believed to release negative ions, which help clear the air of everything from smells to mould spores and bacteria. Since the negative ions are the same as those produced in nature, smoke cleansing can have benefits similar to a walk in the woods.

WHAT YOU NEED

- Dried herbs or plants (try drying your own by tying them together and hanging them upside down in a dry, dark space).

- An abalone shell or other fireproof surface.

- Matches or a lighter.

- A feather (optional).

WHAT TO DO

- Start by lighting your herb bundle and blowing out the flame, just like you would with an incense stick. Using your feather, if you have one, or just your palm, direct the smoke all over your body, closing your eyes if you wish.

- Next, focus on your home, gently waving the smoke into the air and walking from room to room. Pay particular attention to corners and wardrobes. When you're done, allow your herb bundle to burn out on the shell or other fireproof surface.

- Some people go through this ritual with great attention to every aspect of their home once a month or so, but you can give yourself the gift of relaxation by smoke cleansing for just a couple of minutes every morning.

Choosing your herbs

Purifying: chamomile or lemongrass

Healing: amaranth or palo santo

Power and confidence: bay leaf or cedar

Spiritualism vs commercialism

You may have heard of smudging, a Native American ritual practice that is sacred and attached to a range of spiritual beliefs. Smudging bears a resemblance to smoke cleansing, but the commercial products that have recently become popular throughout the West do not necessarily represent the values and spiritual depth of the practice of these indigenous groups. Therefore, it's important to remember to treat the practice with respect. And if you enjoy smoke cleansing, you could perhaps read up on your own culture's old herb-burning traditions, which were more widespread than most people realize.

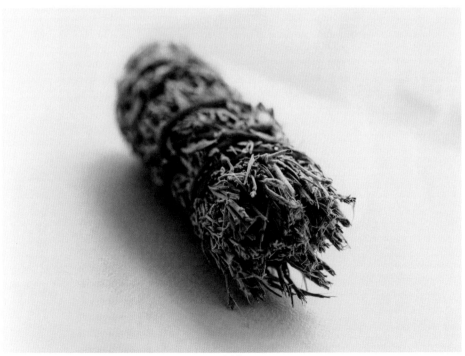

WEEKEND CLEANSING RITUAL: CREATE A HOME SPA

If you feel limited in terms of what you have time for on a weekday morning, make the most of the space of weekend mornings, or whichever days your schedule allows. A home spa can be as spartan or indulgent as you like, with strict Ayurvedic treatments or rose petals and manicures galore. Listen to what your body needs, and then let your creativity run wild.

THE ULTIMATE SEVEN-STEP SOAK

1. For a slow but pampering, rehydrating bath ritual, fill a hot bath, adding a drop of lavender essential oil, and light a few scented candles or some incense if that helps you to relax. Perhaps make a cup of herbal tea and put on some calming music.

2. Before you get in the bath, prepare your skin with a facial steam. Just fill a bowl with hot water and a ripped-open herbal tea bag, and then lean over the bowl with a towel over your head. Breathe slowly for 5–10 minutes.

3. All steamed and ready, get into the bath and treat yourself to a nourishing hair mask. You can make your own by simply whisking together 1 egg yolk, 2 tablespoons coconut oil and 1 tablespoon honey. Leave it in for around half an hour, during which time you can apply a face mask of your choice (see page 140).

Continued overleaf

Try dry brushing

As the name suggests, dry brushing is best done on dry skin; however, you can use a scented body oil, if you prefer.

Using a skin brush, start at your feet and brush up toward the heart, using either small, firm upward strokes or circular motions. On your stomach, use anticlockwise strokes.

Brush for a minimum of 3 minutes.

A word on essential oils

Essential oils can be incredibly powerful, so be careful when experimenting with them and never use them undiluted. For topical application, a two percent dilution is usually recommended for safe home practice. A good rule of thumb is to mix 12 drops of essential oil with 30ml (1fl oz) of carrier oil (such as almond oil) or moisturizer.

Be sure to perform a patch test before using it. To do this, blend a drop of essential oil with 1 teaspoon olive oil, put a few drops of the diluted oil on a plaster or bandage and apply it to the inside of your arm. If no irritation arises within 48 hours, you are safe to proceed with using the oil.

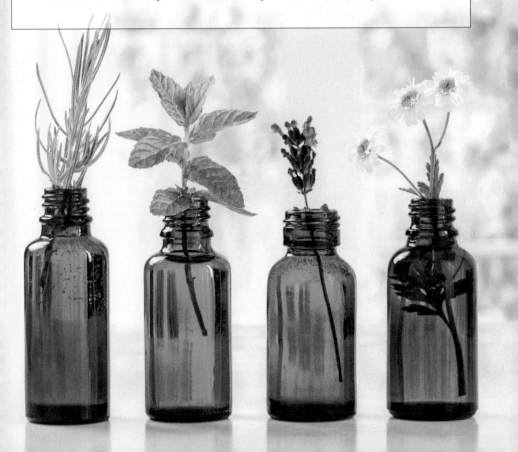

Spirulina face mask

FOR REDUCING REDNESS

Take a small bowl, add 2 tablespoons spirulina powder and a few drops of water; stir to combine into a paste. Apply to your face, leave to dry and wait 20 minutes before you wipe it off with a warm, wet face towel.

Bicarbonate of soda face mask

*FOR DEEP-CLEANSING AND
REDUCING INFLAMMATION*

Mix equal parts bicarbonate of soda (baking soda) and water or apple cider vinegar. Add a drop of essential oil, if you wish and you know that your skin can cope with it (see page 139). Rub into the skin with circular motions and leave for a few minutes before rinsing with warm water.

Essential beard oil

FOR GENERAL BEARD MAINTENANCE

Blend a couple of drops of eucalyptus or cedarwood essential oil with roughly 2 tablespoons olive oil or coconut oil, and massage into your beard. Many people swear by their chosen combination of oils for faster growth and a thicker beard, and while there is mainly only anecdotal evidence to back up such claims, an oil mask will certainly help with rehydration and a healthy glow.

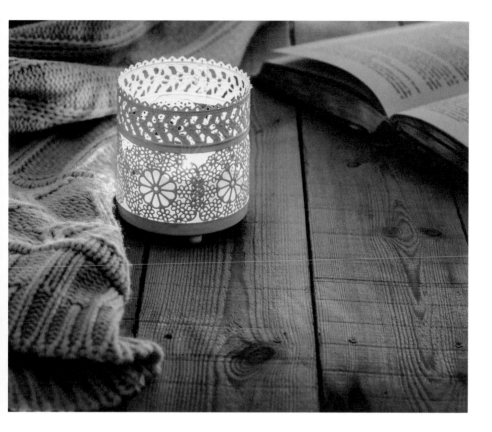

4. Give yourself a relaxing oil massage or foot scrub and rub, or just soak in the bath and breathe. Soon, just the scent of lavender on any given morning will make your shoulders drop and forehead relax.

5. Take the time to dry yourself properly, rubbing the skin all over to remove any dead skin cells. Then moisturize with a body butter or oil, paying attention to everything from your cuticles to your lower back.

6. Rehydrate inside and out: drink a large glass of water and apply toner to your face – a mix of one part apple cider vinegar to four parts water makes a refreshing skin toner.

7. Next? Get ready, perhaps make brunch, and enjoy your weekend smelling lovely and with an unmistakable glow.

IF YOU ONLY DO ONE THING...
Whether your morning facial cleansing routine is a quick rinse and rehydration fix or you go through an elaborate procedure of scrubbing, toning, oiling and more, try committing to it with a little extra self-care, whether by lighting a scented candle or by giving yourself a gentle face massage. It won't necessarily require more time – just a moment's awareness.

CLEANSE – SUGGESTED RITUALS
Start the day with a true act of self-care

A full-body cleanse doesn't have to be time-consuming and a little bit of spa luxury doesn't need to be complicated. Inspired by these rituals, you can start your day by treating your body, be it with a quick but loving touch or with all the wisdom of Ayurveda.

RITUAL FOR THE TIME-POOR

– Rise early.

– Burn some incense and dry brush your body (see page 138), from the feet up, for a total of 3–4 minutes.

– Have a shower, brush your teeth and scrape your tongue (see page 132).

– Make sure to rehydrate your skin, especially on your face, with your choice of moisturizer or oil.

– Get dressed and ready, grabbing an egg and some nuts or a chia pudding (see page 114) to enjoy on the go – unless you choose to leave breakfast for a little later.

RITUAL FOR THE TIME-RICH

– Rise before dawn, as prescribed by Ayurvedic thought (see page 128).

– Practise some *kapalabhati* breathing (see page 39) followed by a few minutes of sitting in silence.

– Pamper your body with a treatment suited to that day: soak in a hot bath if you are not on a deadline; oil your body if you're feeling a little cold and in need of a gentle massage (see page 135); or apply a home-made face mask to give your face that lift (see page 140).

– Meditate (see page 42) as you wait for the face mask to do its magic.

– Dry yourself, get dressed and enjoy a fruit or veg shake (see page 115), perhaps with a superfood or two mixed in (see page 112).

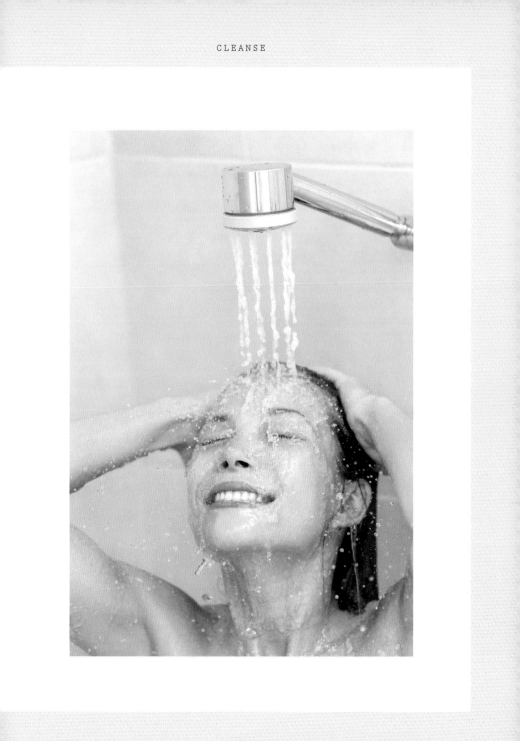

"Nothing is more beautiful
than the loveliness of the
woods before sunrise."
— GEORGE WASHINGTON CARVER

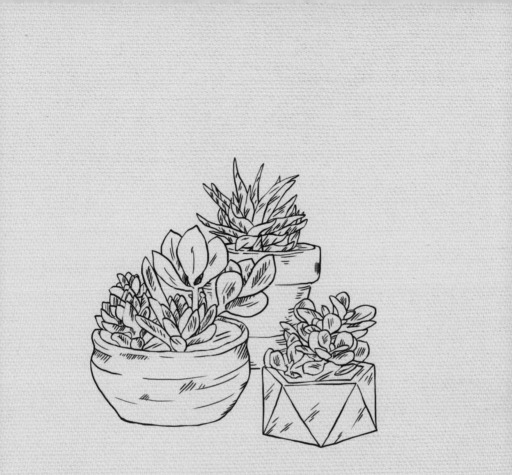

CHAPTER 7

CONNECT

Rituals in nature

"One touch of nature makes
the whole world kin."
— WILLIAM SHAKESPEARE

THE POWER
OF NATURE

Every time I arrive somewhere by the sea, I am overwhelmed by acute euphoria, a kind of blissful gratitude that I can't put into words. I've recently become aware that I'm not alone – the sea seems to have that effect on people. In fact, much of nature seems to produce in us a sense of wonder, a sudden awareness that we are part of something greater than we can comprehend. That's no mean feat in a world where many people are feeling increasingly lonely and disillusioned.

MAGNIFICENT SILENCE

The peacefulness that envelops you as you stroll through nature without headphones is not a deafening silence. In some ways, it is more like nature's own wonderfully tumultuous anarchy. It is busy, ever-changing and unpredictable – but not in the overwhelming way of social media's bombardment of change and uncertainty. No, this is the peacefully multifaceted patchwork of nature that makes us feel tiny yet connected, not by "friend" requests but by beautiful necessity. It is the grounding reminder that we are part of something bigger.

AT ONE WITH THE EARTH

For many people, a morning ritual is all about being fully present in the moment, rejecting fears and stressful thoughts. Walking barefoot through grass, paying attention to early birdsong or, indeed, spending time by the sea is an ideal way to heighten that experience. It takes time to master the art of being present with nothing but your breath, but when surrounded by the extraordinary changeability of nature, you are almost immediately drawn back into the present moment, your breath at one with the pulse of the earth.

GETTING OUT THERE

There are endless ways to bring a little bit of nature into your morning ritual. It doesn't need to involve going for a run or throwing yourself into the ice-cold sea – though it certainly can. Getting a dog, which will have to be walked in all weathers, is another way to ensure you spend more time in nature. Plus, owning a dog is a proven way to boost happiness. Just start by opening up that back door, kicking your slippers off and stepping outside.

NATURAL PANACEA

Look to science and you will find that nature is something of a super-drug. Simply being in it reduces anxiety and the production of stress hormones, lowers your blood pressure and heart rate, helps decrease the levels of inflammation in the body and boosts the amount of oxygen transported around your bloodstream, providing increased clarity and focus.

MOTHER NATURE AT HER BEST

A good dose of vitamin D from sunshine exposure has countless health benefits: it helps your bones develop properly and can reduce the risk of multiple sclerosis, diabetes and metabolic syndrome. Moreover, exposure to daylight can boost your melatonin levels at night, giving you a better night's sleep. Yes, studies have shown that living near green areas gives you a greater shot at a longer life, but simply getting closer to nature, wherever you are, boosts happiness.

AWESOME HEALING

One of many reasons why spending time in nature has a relaxing effect and helps reduce stress levels is the very mechanism by which trees and plants protect themselves from insects and rot. They emit chemicals, sometimes referred to as wood essential oils, that linger in the forest air – chemicals that, among other things, have a calming effect and impact positively on so-called natural killer cells in our immune system. So, the by-product of trees' self-protection becomes a healing gift for us humans. Truly awe-inspiring.

Being surrounded by life is, in itself, life-affirming; the experience of the vitality of nature helps awaken your senses and breathe energy into your soul. That euphoria upon arriving by the sea that I mentioned on page 147 is a prime example of what researchers call an increased sense of awe, something that enhances life satisfaction and contributes to a drop in markers of inflammation. (Although inflammation is an integral part of the body's healing process, it is also easily triggered by diet and lifestyle choices and is a contributing factor behind many chronic diseases.)

"To sit in the shade on a
fine day and look upon verdure
is the most perfect refreshment."
— JANE AUSTEN

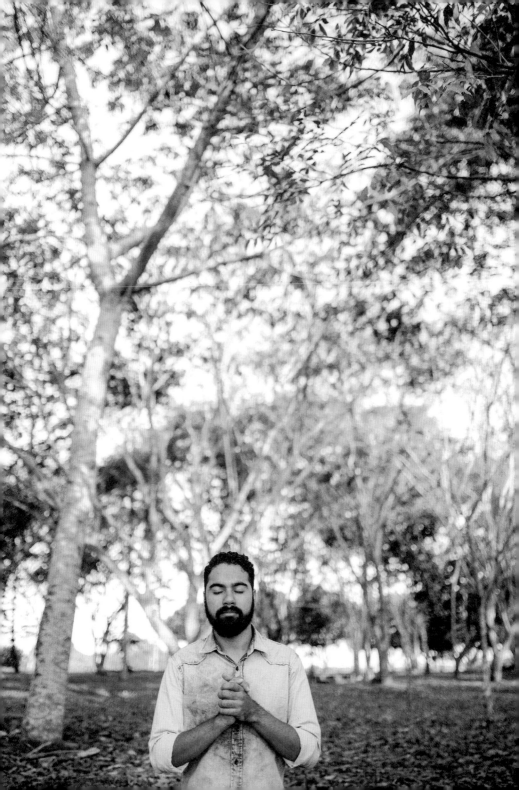

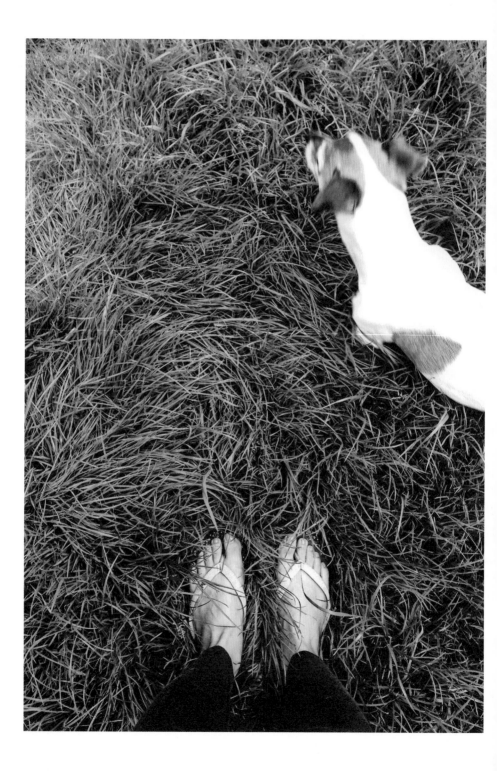

GREENIFY
YOUR MORNING

If you like the sound of incorporating nature into your morning routine but don't quite know where to start, here are a few ideas to inspire you.

EXERCISE OUTDOORS

Outdoor exercise boosts your mood and self-esteem in as little as 5 minutes and, of course, exercise of any kind brings a long list of very attractive benefits. Why not go running or cycling or do some yoga in the park?

WATCH THE SUNRISE

Get comfortable with your favourite blanket and a cup of tea on your balcony or porch, or pick a well-positioned bench in the local park, and watch the beauty of nature unfold. Just looking at nature, research shows, increases your ability to concentrate. Moments of mindfulness don't come much better than this.

GROUP WORKOUT

Get up close and personal with the elements, regardless of weather, with a group session, be it a neighbourhood jogging club or an army boot camp. The community spirit usually brings added motivation and you'll feel like a winner before the day has even really begun.

MEDITATION OR BREATHING

Many people find meditating easier outside in nature, as the sounds are often soothing and less distracting. Focus on your breath and feel how it moves with nature with the wind and the trees.

MINDFUL WALK

Stroll through your garden or the streets of your neighbourhood – observe the changes of the seasons, listen to birdsong, notice what the breeze feels like on your skin and how the light changes every day. Activating all your senses helps you to be fully present. Stroll barefoot through grass or lean against a big, old tree to feel extra grounded.

GO FOR A SWIM

Whether in the sea, a nearby lake or the local pond or swimming pool, a morning dip can be hugely refreshing and life-affirming. Find a morning swimming group (see page 78) and you might make friends for life.

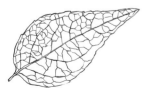

GET IN THE SEA – SAFELY

Sea swimming can be deeply invigorating, not to mention the additional benefits if you found your own local swim collective. Former British Champion surfer, environmentalist and keen swimmer Sophie Hellyer did exactly that when she started the Rise Fierce movement on the Irish Atlantic coast. Here are her tips for staying safe in those wild waves.

TIPS FOR NOVICE SWIMMERS

- Outdoor swimming in cold water saps your body heat, so your arms and legs quickly become weak. This could get you into trouble if you're unable to get out of the water. Wear a wetsuit for anything more than a quick dip. The Rise Fierce crew only gets in for 2–5 minutes when it's cold, and up to 25 minutes in the summer months.

- Make sure you understand the tides, rips, currents and waves where you are swimming. If you're unsure, ask someone more experienced.

- Don't jump into cold water – wade in slowly instead.

- Never go alone. Always swim with a friend or two.

- Swim close to the shore. If it's rough, swim parallel to the shore, well within your depth.

- Shivering and teeth chattering are the first symptoms of hypothermia. If that happens, get out of the water and warm up.

- Take warm clothes to put on afterward – even in summer; you'll feel colder when you get out.

"The man who is swimming against the stream knows the strength of it."
— WOODROW WILSON

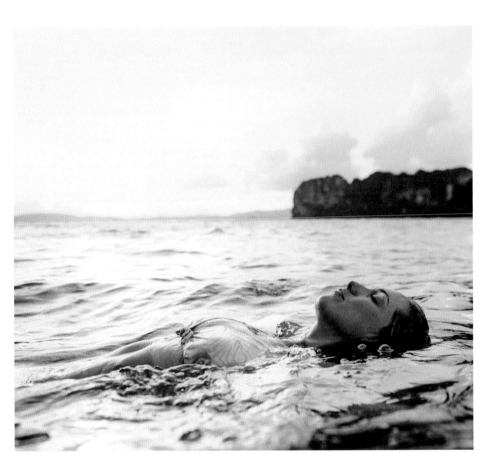

Think of the benefits

Whether in the form of an ice-cold shower or a dip in
the sea, cold-water immersion has many benefits, including
effective pain relief and soothing muscle aches. It has also
been proven to boost your immune system, increase dopamine
levels and help with managing anxiety.

BRING NATURE INSIDE

---

*To some, a morning in nature sounds lovely in theory
but gets tricky when the reality of life kicks in -
perhaps especially for single parents, who can't
just hop into running shoes and walk out the door.*

However, multiple studies show that you can reap some of the benefits of time in nature just by looking at photos of it or bringing it inside. One study from Kansas State University looked at patients recovering from surgery and found that those in rooms with plants did better than those in rooms without, in terms of everything from blood pressure to anxiety and pain levels. Other studies have concluded that just looking at a video of nature scenes can speed up recovery from stress, while visualizing or looking at pictures of nature tends to boost energy levels.

WHAT CAN YOU DO?

- Do you have indoor plants? Water them, chat to them, give them a shower in the bathtub occasionally – and invest in some more. They add character to a space, kids can have great fun looking after them and watching them grow, and the plants are bound to purify both the air and a little part of your soul.

- If you like the idea of a vision board (see page 58), create one inspired by nature. It doesn't have to be all green; there are plants and flowers in every colour of the rainbow. Speaking of which, you can always include a rainbow, the moon and the stars. The sky is the limit, almost literally.

- Do you have a home altar (see page 165), perhaps with candles or incense? It's the ideal place to add some pine cones, colourful leaves or branches, or perhaps a few shells from the beach. If a home altar is not your thing, a nature table works, too. Spend a moment by it every morning, perhaps rearranging a few stones or tending to your succulents. Whenever there is time, go for a morning stroll through your local park and replace a few items on the home altar or nature table to reflect the changing seasons.

IF YOU ONLY DO ONE THING...

You might not be ready to leave the house every morning before you shower and have breakfast, but try spending a few minutes drinking your morning beverage of choice sitting in the doorway, on the balcony or in the garden, just taking in your surroundings, listening to birdsong and watching your neighbourhood wake up.

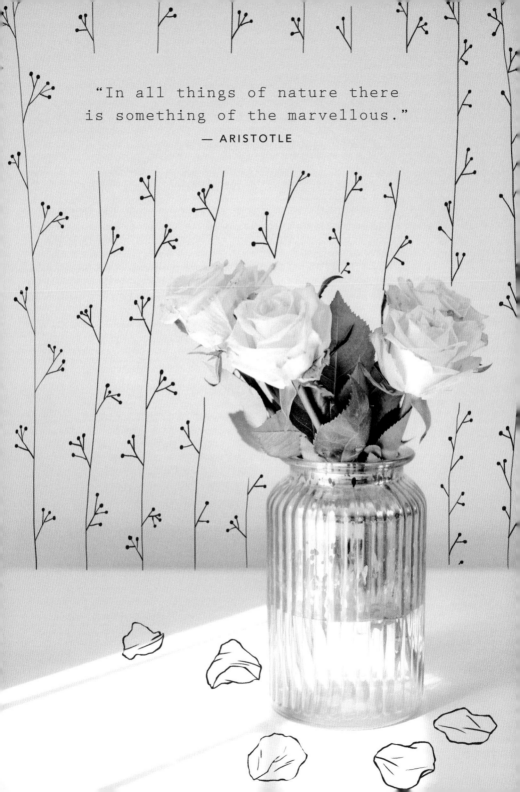

"In all things of nature there is something of the marvellous."
— ARISTOTLE

CONNECT – SUGGESTED RITUALS

Wake up and feel part of a beautiful greater whole

Nature on its own can be the greatest medicine. Combined with elements of other rituals, it can be a priceless mood booster. These suggested rituals can be tweaked to suit your location and available amenities; see them as a jumping-off point, then get creative with whatever nature has to offer where you are.

RITUAL FOR THE TIME-POOR

– Rise, shower and get dressed, checking in with yourself and your wardrobe list of core values (see page 96).

– Open up the back door or a window to let in some fresh air. Allow yourself to pay attention to the smells and sounds of nature as you make yourself a grate-and-infuse drink (see page 119).

– Grab an egg or a pre-prepared chia pudding (see page 114), and check in on your plants – talking to them is perfectly acceptable, even recommended!

– Cycle to work, and opt for the scenic route through the park or along the canal towpath.

RITUAL FOR THE TIME-RICH

– Rise at dawn.

– Wrap up, take a stroll through the neighbourhood or local park, and take a few deep breaths.

– Be mindful of the sounds of nature, the feeling of the breeze on your face, how the light changes as the sun rises; if you have a nature table or corner at home, perhaps collect a particularly beautiful leaf to take home with you.

– Visit a nearby lake, lido or the sea for a morning dip.

– When you get home, enjoy a hot drink on the balcony or by the window as you list, even just mentally, a few things you are grateful for.

– Shower and get ready for the day ahead.

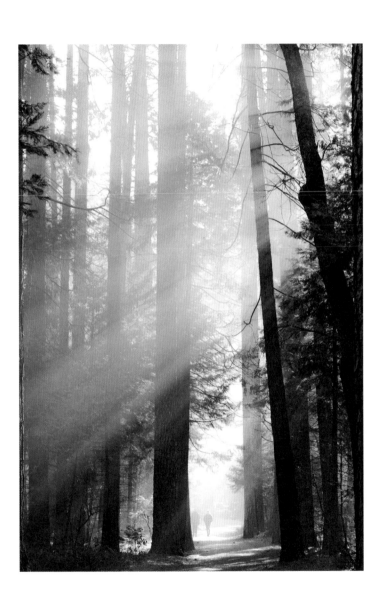

"It is easier to make our wishes
conform to our means than to make
our means conform to our wishes."
— ROBERT E LEE

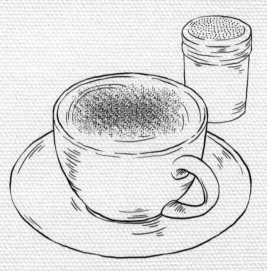

CHAPTER 8

ACCEPT

When life gets in the way

STRIKING THE BALANCE BETWEEN SELF-CONTROL AND ACCEPTANCE

A few months before starting to write this book, I took up daily yoga. I was at the tail end of a years-long, intense project and was exhausted and empty; I was craving self-care more than ever before. My daily yoga sessions, while often short and gentle, became highly addictive very quickly and, a few weeks in, I started mixing the yoga with running and other forms of exercise. The affirmation that I am a person who exercises daily became like a mantra for me, and I felt happier and more grounded than I had in a long time.

WHEN LIFE GETS IN THE WAY

Then I fell ill. It was nothing major – but I couldn't get over the frustration of not being able to get my daily endorphin boost. In my head, my newfound peace of mind was so closely connected to the experience of exercising that I couldn't seem to access it at all when the circumstances changed. My caring for myself had become conditional on my ability to exercise in a certain way, and when I couldn't, I felt only one thing: stress.

FLEXIBLE SELF-CARE

We find something that works for us, we are ecstatic, we want to tell the world about it – and then we feel depressed and hard done by when it's taken away from us. It's hardly surprising. But when a self-care ritual becomes another item on a to-do list, it's time to think again. It's not self-care if you can turn it into a stick to beat yourself with.

PRACTISE ACCEPTANCE

There will be times when illness strikes, your child won't sleep, the housemates are in the way or a new schedule at work turns the day upside-down. You need to be able to find the time and space for a little bit of self-love, without that simply adding to an already stressful situation. And you need to be able to accept those times when you try but fail, rather than beating yourself up about it.

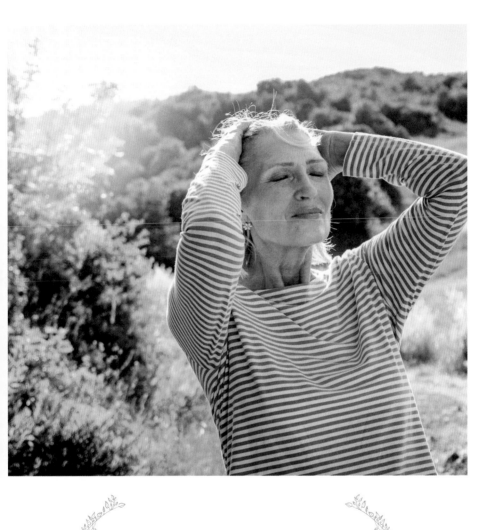

"However long the night,
the dawn will always break."
— AFRICAN PROVERB

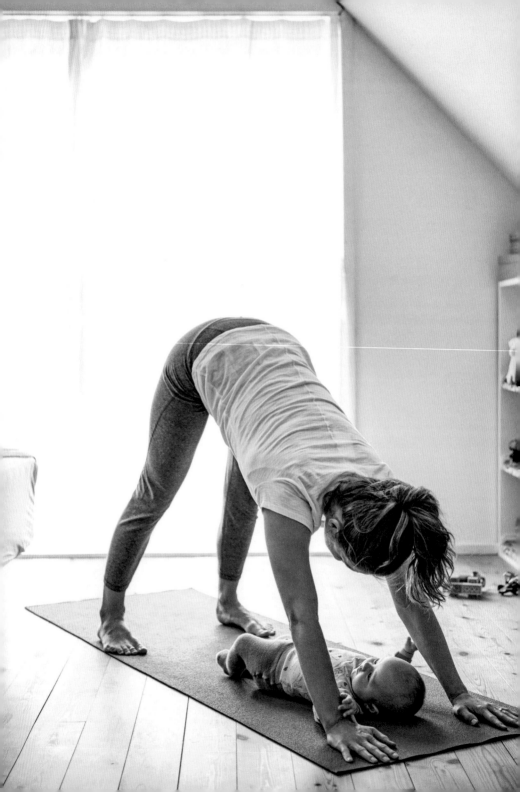

WHAT PARENTS DO

Much of the beauty of rising early is in the experience of that sleepiness, a peacefully quiet world that is almost perfectly still. But add babies and young children to the picture, and it changes drastically. There's nothing peaceful about being woken at dawn by a pile of books dropped onto your face by a toddler who wants to be read a morning story, or the young siblings who can't wait to start playing with their building blocks but just need your help to make toast first.

Ironically, self-care is probably never as badly needed as during those early parenting years, when you've gone from feeling on top of the world to being bottom of the list, always worrying about and caring for other little people, on nowhere near enough sleep and under too much external scrutiny. Though it might seem impossible, some parents have found simple but creative ways to fit in that little bit of morning peace.

TIPS FOR PARENTS

- Get your yoga on – and bring the children along. It won't be the same, and you might not make it all the way to self-realization, but you can definitely get the benefit of a few stretches and keep up that good habit. YouTube channels such as Cosmic Yoga and Yoga Ed. are good places to start, although they are a tad less harmonious than their adult counterparts.

- Mindfulness colouring books started to pop up everywhere a while back, and they provide the perfect opportunity to engage in a creative activity with your little ones over that morning cup of coffee. Ideally, the children will stick to their favourite colouring books and you can keep yours neat and truly mindful, but colouring of any kind lends itself well to a peaceful morning moment.

- Sprinkle some cinnamon onto your morning coffee and set an intention for the day ahead. If you can't find a moment to yourself, tell your children about your intention in words they understand, and invite them to share their hopes for the day as well.

- Whether it is while cosy in bed together just after you wake up, or while having breakfast or reading a morning book on the couch, take a moment to tell your child about something you are grateful for – or, in their words, something that makes you feel good or happy. Then ask them what makes them feel good. This not only brings that abundance mindset (see page 92) to your morning, but also gives your child the gift of a habitual positive outlook.

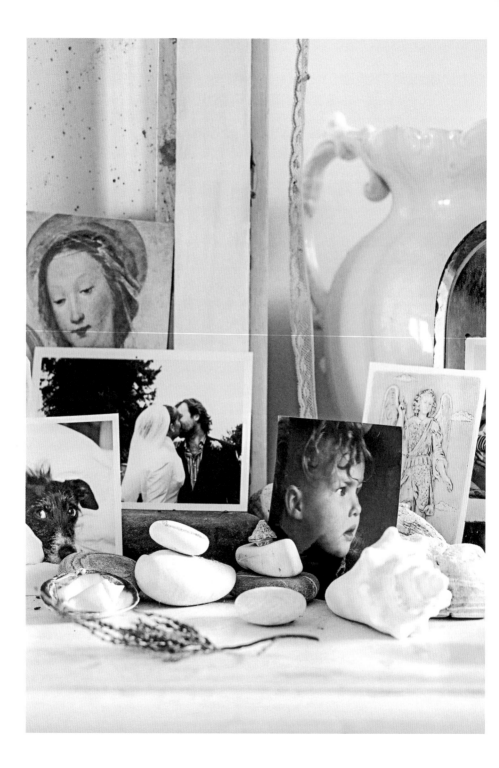

FINDING SPACE WHERE THERE IS NONE

Perhaps you're in a house-share and the only space you can control is one small room, or you're co-sleeping with a baby who nurses all morning. Physical space and privacy are not to be taken for granted, but there are ways to find mental space or a sacred corner of your own in which to ground yourself, no matter where you are. Here are four of them.

1. IF YOU ARE STUCK IN BED
Take a moment to: spot three things you can see; notice three sensations in your body; listen to three sounds you can hear; find three things within arm's reach that you can touch. Fully waking up your senses will bring you straight into the present moment.

2. AS YOU GET OUT OF BED
Enjoy a full-body stretch, reaching for the ceiling and feeling how the spine stretches out, one vertebra at a time. Take a deep breath in, exhale fully and, if you like, say an affirmation or set an intention for the day.

3. CREATE A HOME ALTAR
Use religious symbols for a moment of morning prayer or photographs of loved ones, memorabilia and candles. It can be a little arrangement on your bedside table, on a dressing table or on a small shelf. If you don't pray, simply enjoy a moment of mindfulness at your home altar before you get ready for the day ahead.

4. FIND INSPIRATION
Read about the mini rituals for the brain on page 96 for some more inspiration on simple ways to find mental peace and space.

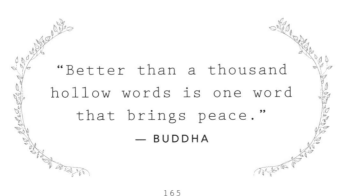

"Better than a thousand hollow words is one word that brings peace."
— BUDDHA

Living with illness

Different obstacles present different challenges and sometimes
physical or mental illness can make finding a morning ritual
just as tricky as limited time and space. I've come across
mothers of severely disabled children who are full-time carers
and have made a habit of rising before dawn to write because
the world they create in their stories is the only real break
they get. I've spoken to those living with chronic pain who
cope thanks to a morning ritual of meditation and the Chinese
martial art T'ai Chi. No one knows your particular situation
better than you do, but working with it is likely to be far
healthier and more effective than trying to work against it.

When grief strikes

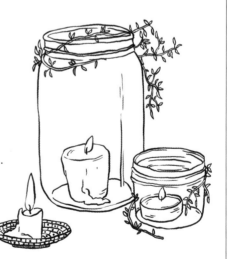

On life's darkest days,
acknowledging your feelings
can be more important than
searching for the gratitude
within. Looking at a photo
of a person you've lost and
lighting a candle can be a
beautiful, if heart-breaking,
way to be with and honour them.

WHEN ALL ELSE FAILS

A few of the people I've interviewed for this book have spoken about their morning ritual helping them to feel in control. Let's not confuse this with being in control. You can feel in control in the sense that you are focused and grounded and capable of dealing with whatever the day throws at you - but you can't control whether that will be eggs or rose petals, good news or devastating phone calls. Accepting that is an important first step in letting go of expectations that will likely lead to disappointment sooner or later.

ACCEPTANCE AS THE FIRST STEP TO SELF-CARE

Stepping onto the yoga mat is your victory; your body falling apart or the house burning down is beyond your control. Putting on your running shoes and striding out the door is your act of self-care; you can't stop a hurricane while you're running. Sitting down, pen in hand, is showing commitment; if 5 minutes later you're stuck for words or the ink runs out, that's not to say that you failed. The next day, you try again.

YES, LIFE WILL GET IN THE WAY

Even the most dedicated yogis have times when they can't get to the mat. For sure, there are days when journal pages are left empty and incense sticks remain untouched. If you have a desire to make the most of that morning magic, you will do so when things settle. In the meantime, remember that self-judgment won't get you there.

UPSIDE-DOWN SCHEDULES

Many workers will be familiar with rising at different, sometimes awkward times, which means that committing to a ritual at a set time every day might seem impossible. Some choose to have their moment when they rise, whatever time of day or night that is; others make a habit out of taking a 5-minute break at around the same time every day, even if they are at work. Advanced rituals may go out the window, but your breath and awareness are always with you. By embracing some of the ideas on page 168, you should soon find that ritual needn't be entirely impossible, no matter how demanding your schedule.

IF YOU ONLY DO ONE THING...

Forget rules and promises, including everything you ever thought a morning ritual has to be. Have a cry if you need to, go back to sleep, cuddle your kids or call a friend for a chat – whatever acceptance of the situation looks like to you. Even with a long-established morning ritual, there will be days like these. If today you accept that, that's a victory in itself.

Ritual for those with tricky schedules

Do you rise at different or awkward times? Perhaps you travel a lot and your internal body clock is confused? Try to separate the idea of getting out of bed from that of your morning ritual.

1. When you have your first tea or coffee of the day, wherever you are and whatever time it is, make sure to get some space, switch off your phone and take 5 minutes to think about what you are grateful for. Commit to this every day and you will soon find that there's a nice, familiar rhythm to it - even if the clock does not agree.

2. Afterward, or as soon as your schedule allows, do a full-body stretch. As you reach for the sky, take a deep breath and, on the exhale, set an intention for the day (see page 57).

3. Incorporate your own, personalized elements to this ritual: you might draw a daily oracle card (also know as wisdom or tarot cards), pray in the same place every day or jot down goals or tasks whenever you find the time. It's your commitment that matters - not what it looks like.

"Because one believes in oneself, one doesn't try to convince others. Because one is content with oneself, one doesn't need others' approval. Because one accepts oneself, the whole world accepts him or her."

— LAO TZU

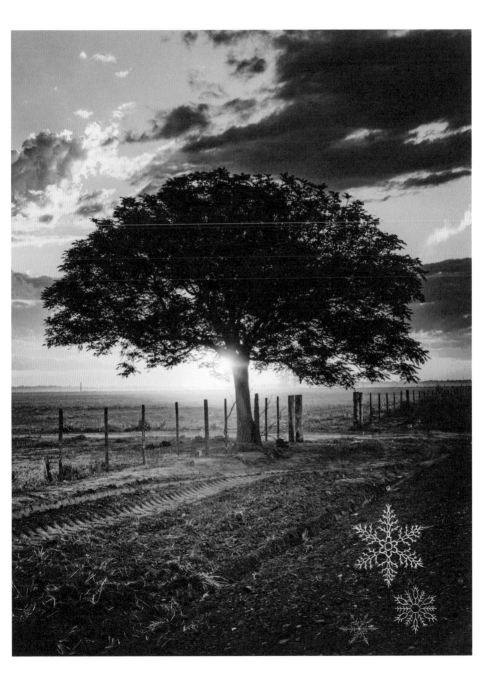

ACCEPT – SUGGESTED RITUALS

Steeped in self-kindness, it becomes easier to try - even when you fail

---

Awkward work schedules, tricky home situations and a lack of space are all reasons why adopting a morning ritual can prove difficult - and why some never bother trying. Apply a healthy dose of flexibility and self-kindness, and one of these suggested rituals might inspire you to try with an open mind...

RITUAL FOR
STAY-AT-HOME PARENTS

– Rise with the kids – that's probably early enough.

– Feed everyone what they need to avoid hunger-related chaos, be that a banana or a full breakfast spread.

– Prepare a hot drink of your choice, perhaps warm lemon (see page 110).

– Get out colouring books, sheets of paper, crayons and pens. Either doodle together or let the kids do their thing while you do some mindful colouring.

– Take a moment for yourself whenever you can, perhaps to sprinkle some cinnamon into your coffee, or maybe just open up the back door or a window for some fresh air, and think about what matters most to you today.

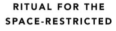

RITUAL FOR THE
SPACE-RESTRICTED

– Wake up early – before the others in the house, if you can, especially if you are in a house share.

– Practise some in-bed morning yoga (see page 50).

– Get cosy sitting up in bed, and do some bullet journalling (see page 89) or write down a handful of things you are grateful for (see page 91).

– Get up, head to the bathroom and wake up your face and eyes with an Ayurvedic rinse (see page 131).

– Enjoy a bowl of overnight oats (see page 115), or, if it's the weekend, why not surprise your housemates with some freshly baked bread (see page 117), if your kitchen space allows?

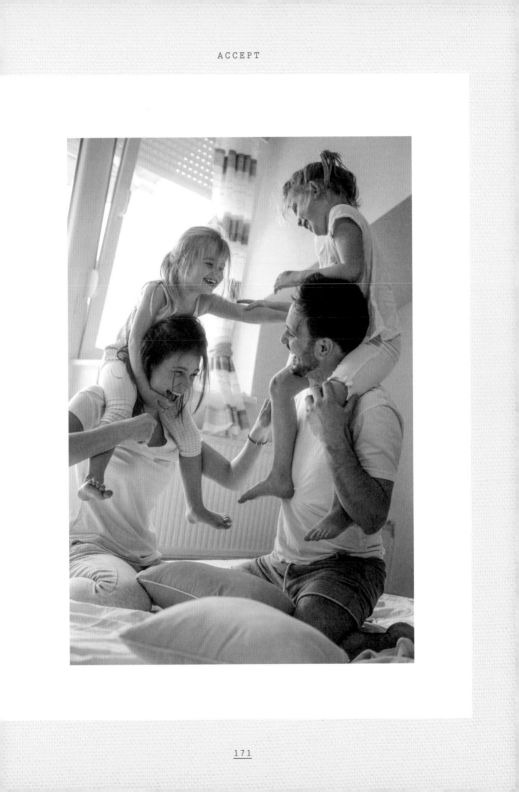

"The breeze at dawn has
secrets to tell you.
Don't go back to sleep."

— RUMI

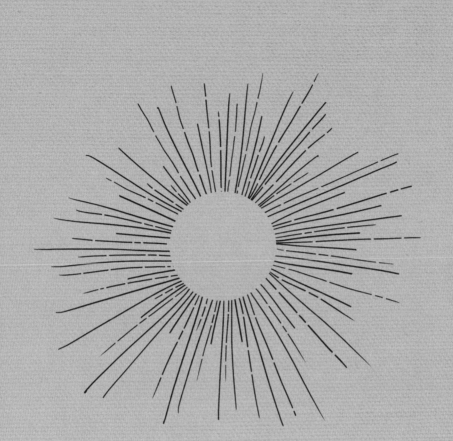

CHAPTER 9

TRUST

Finding your flow

WHAT DOES YOUR IDEAL DAY LOOK LIKE?

Close your eyes. Take a deep breath. Now imagine waking up to your ideal morning. What does it feel like? Where are you? Imagine what it looks like as the morning light enters the window. Do the curtains flutter? Perhaps you're outside, watering roses in a lush garden, or maybe it is still dark, with a big, old floor lamp lighting up the room where a beautiful notebook lies open on a new page.

GO ON, KEEP IMAGINING

Think about what you're wearing, what the clothes feel like. Picture your home, imagine the sounds and smells and then begin to watch the day unfold: where you work; whether you have anyone to say goodbye to before you go; how you feel as you set about your day.

A lasting morning ritual is never just a means to an end, never just a thing to get through; it is part of a journey you want to be on right now, woven into the fabric of your life as you imagine it when you dare to dream.

WHAT COMES FIRST, THE RITUAL OR THE DREAM?

Be brave and dare to paint a picture of your ideal scenario. Maybe you have plans for major changes in your life; maybe you are exactly where you want to be, but you'd like to invest more in yourself and your wellbeing. When you visualize your morning at its best, you can discover a good place to start in creating your very own ritual.

"Habit is a cable; we weave a thread of it each day, and at last we cannot break it."
— HORACE MANN

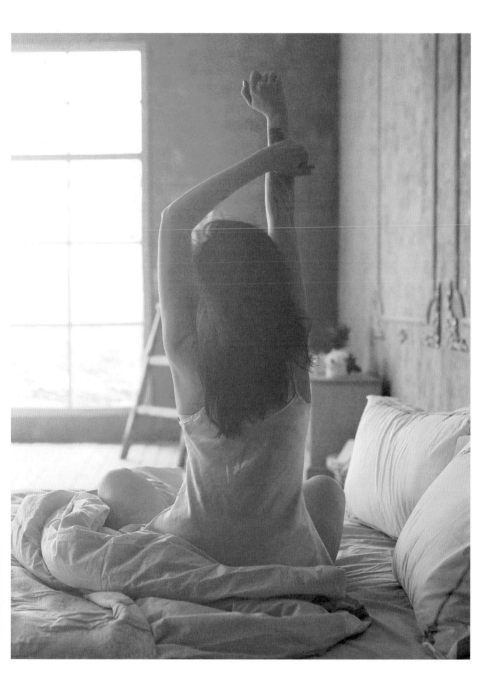

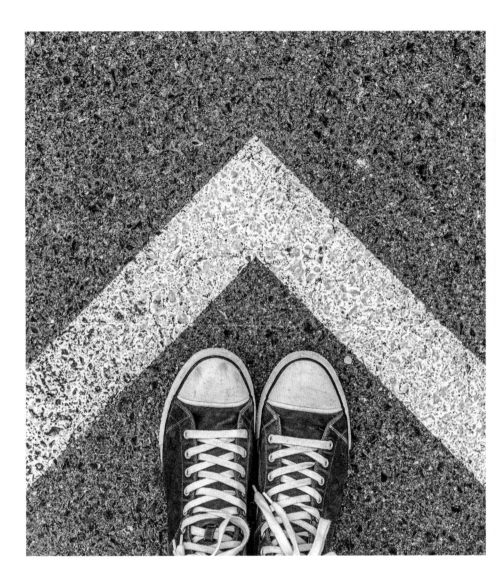

"Man often becomes what he
believes himself to be."

— MAHATMA GANDHI

THINK OUTSIDE THE BOX

If thinking about your ideal morning makes you none the wiser, and getting started with designing a morning ritual from scratch seems like an impossible task, shaking things up with a different perspective and some inspiration from those you admire most might help.

BE INSPIRED BY YOUR ROLE MODELS

I had a role model once. A highly unlikely one. She was a fashion icon and a real business head; I was known for having a strong dislike of both of those things. So why did I look up to her? Because of how she was: how she spoke to people, her integrity and her tireless dedication.

Take a leaf out of the productivity books that suggest you look to your role models for guidance – and do so when thinking about what you want from a morning ritual. List your role models, describe in detail what you admire about them and find the common denominators. If your role models all exude strength and determination, then think about how you might start your day to feed those traits in yourself.

BREAK YOUR PATTERN

If you're a writer, it might be tempting to start the day with journalling or stream-of-consciousness writing, but is that really going to add much to your day? Similarly, to a project manager, to-do lists and goal setting probably won't feel a lot like self-care, while carers might want a break from oils and creams. It could be better for you to try something completely new.

However different all the aspects of a morning ritual covered in this book may be, they have this in common: they promote awareness and consciousness over unthinking, unconscious habits. Even goal setting and guided visualization, while sometimes working with a vision of something quite different from the present, provide the mental clarity and focus that help bring you back to yourself and what's going on right now. See what happens when you challenge yourself to step out of your comfort zone. Sometimes a little bit of change and a different perspective are all you need.

QUESTIONS TO ASK YOURSELF

*Your morning ritual needs to be unique to you, so who better
to ask about the intricacies of the vision you wish to create?*

- How do you want to feel by the end of your morning ritual? Focused and determined, or calm and open? Buzzed-up and strong, or rested and at peace?

- Are there circumstances, such as illnesses and disabilities, spatial aspects, time pressures or other commitments, that will determine what you can or can't do?

- Are there types of morning rituals that put you off? If so, can you work out why they do and what that tells you?

- What is your main motivation for wanting a morning ritual?

DO SOME BRAINSTORMING

Brainstorm whichever way you prefer to – with a mind map (see box below), lists, a vision board (see page 58) or simply by emptying everything that pops into your mind onto a sheet of paper.

Play around with some ideas or dip in and out of this book, and perhaps try out a few exercises to see how they make you feel.

Remember, you can keep tweaking as your needs and circumstances change. The journey never ends.

Mapping your mind

A mind map is a diagram that visually represents your
thoughts. Simply start with "My Morning" in a circle
at the centre of a blank page, and then draw branches
from that to other circles that contain your thoughts,
ideas, fears or questions. Each of these can have more
sub-branches with related ideas. You can colour-code them
or just write down thoughts without worrying about the
design – whatever helps you to organize your thinking.

"I want to write, but more than that, I want to bring out all kinds of things that lie buried deep in my heart."
— ANNE FRANK

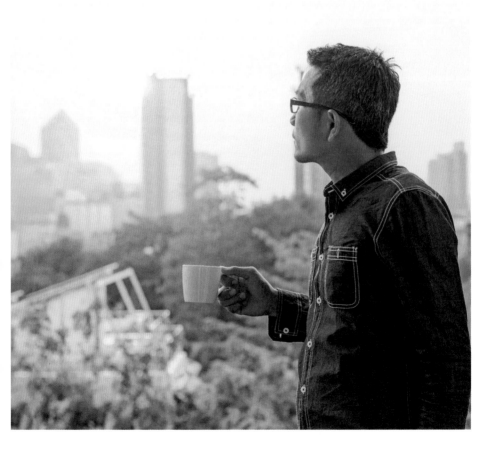

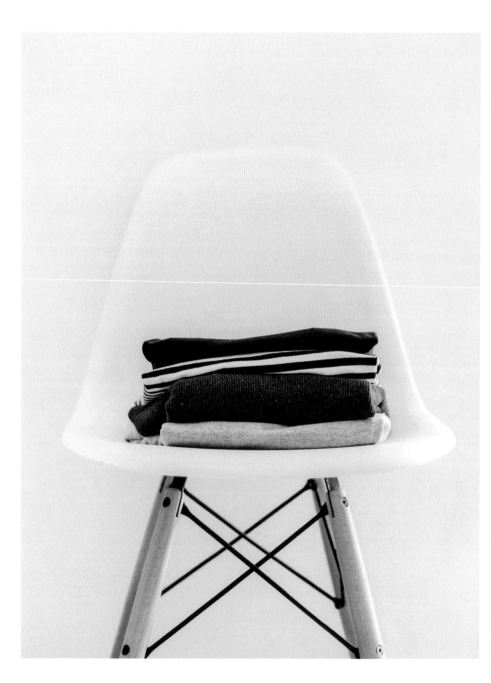

SETTING YOURSELF UP WELL

*To all you fellow night owls out there, I am sorry to bring
you this news: great-quality sleep comes earlier at night.
Some researchers argue that the 3 or 4 hours immediately after
11pm are crucial to a really good night's sleep, while others
say that the ideal bedtime varies from person to person but
that going to bed before midnight is key to waking up rested.
Whatever lights-off time you aim for, planning ahead can
help to minimize friction and avoid unexpected obstacles.*

THINGS TO CONSIDER

- **Breakfast:** Do you have everything you need for your morning tonic or breakfast of choice? You might want to prepare some overnight oats or a chia pudding (see pages 114–15).

- **Clothing:** Leave out the clothes you are going to wear the next day. One decision less in the morning means one more moment's space for yourself.

- **Alarm:** Did you know that there are apps to help you get out of bed? Some require you to scan objects placed throughout your home before they allow you to switch the alarm off, to ensure that you are wide awake and won't go back to bed. If you use your cell phone as your alarm, be sure to pick a sound that is pleasant yet spirited.

- **Devices:** It is obviously difficult to put a curfew on screen time, but you'll find it easier to get to sleep if you haven't just been staring at a bright screen. Find a way to wind down offline before you go to bed.

What's that, an evening ritual?

If you're thriving on the morning ritual, why not create an evening ritual, too? In addition to the things to consider (see left), you could do your gratitude journalling before turning out the lights.

This, in turn, will enable you to incorporate some gratitude into your morning ritual, as you can read through the previous evening's journalling to start the day in a positive way.

WHAT NOT TO DO

While "doing what works" is probably the best piece of advice anyone can give you when it comes to self-care, there are morning habits that have been proven counterproductive and are best avoided.

CHECK YOUR EMAIL

Considering that so many people use their morning ritual as a means to getting one step ahead, it is understandable that it is oh-so-tempting to check your email first thing: to make sure that no catastrophe has erupted overnight, or to quickly reply to one email to show that you are "on it". And some of those big-shot CEOs will admit that they have almost always checked their emails before their morning ritual is over. Nevertheless, it is ill-advised, so much so that entire books have been written on the subject.

Not only does checking your emails first thing trigger "work mode", which leaves little mental space for meditation, but productivity experts have identified another problem with it. Starting by responding to other people's queries gets you into a reactive mode rather than a proactive one; instead of rising early to take control of your day and look inward, you are effectively solving other people's problems at a time when you used to still be in bed. What's the point in rising early for that? Add to that the fact that bad news can hike up your cortisol and adrenaline levels so much that your entire day seems steeped in dread. Obviously there are much better ways to start your day.

Instead... If you like the sound of an action-focused morning, your time is probably better spent identifying the handful of tasks you absolutely have to get done today. Then, once you get to your inbox, your plan is already made and right there waiting for you.

LIGHT A CANDLE

I'm a fan of candles, too, and I love the idea of a tea light or two in the morning, especially in the winter. The bad news is that candlelight will make your body think that it's time to unwind and perhaps even go back to bed.

Instead... If rising early is new to you, you are better off turning the lights on and opening the curtains wide – you can light all the candles you want in the evening.

START WITH COFFEE

It can be tempting, especially if you are not an early bird, to knock back a short black first thing to get that energy boost. Ideally, you should hold off drinking coffee for a little while after you wake up, and certainly avoid drinking caffeine on an empty stomach.

Instead... Start your day with a glass of water to rehydrate (see page 122), or hold off on the coffee until you've had a light breakfast.

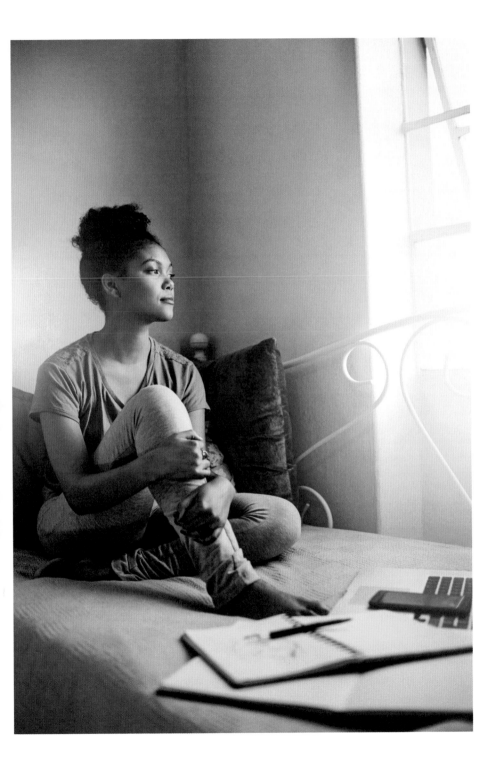

SELF-REALIZATION AND SOVEREIGNTY

Morning rituals are having a moment right now. They've gone from niche productivity circles to the mainstream. But why? Is it simply because we're catching up with an insufficiently conscious lifestyle and with warning signs that are trying to tell us that we need more, and different, care? Or is it because the world feels like it keeps spinning faster and faster, with technological connectivity making us lonelier than ever? If we were always searching for meaning, why were we not all doing this years ago?

While writing this book, I've been thinking a lot about sovereignty: about the state of having sovereign power and authority, of intentional living and being consciously in charge. Self-realization in the spiritual sense, I think, is far removed from self-realization in the eyes of a market-driven culture, and the challenge of inward listening may seem more delicate and complex than ever. Self-care in the age of social media therefore requires digging deeper.

Maybe what is happening right now is that we're urgently yearning for that sovereignty, determined to dig deeper to see what we find when we stop and actually look at the world around us. The way I see it, this isn't a selfish desire, but a responsible reaction to a world in which the pace and noise of living leave little time for reflection and make it hard to listen to each other and ourselves.

The people who are doing this do it because it's too important not to: they want to realize the vision of a lifetime, change their neurological makeup, maybe change the world. What's too important for you to let go of?

Remember, it doesn't matter what your dream is, it just has to be *your* dream.

> "To be yourself in a world that is constantly trying to make you something else is the greatest accomplishment."
>
> — RALPH WALDO EMERSON

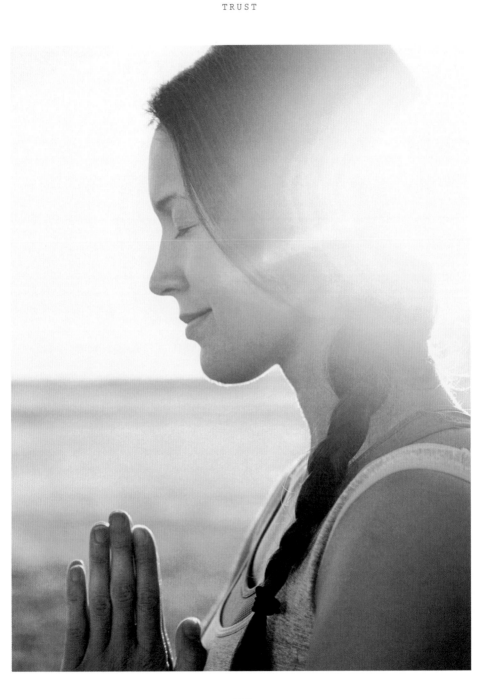

TAKE THIS WITH YOU...

---

*The reason the daily habit works for most people is that,
once you've decided that you're doing this thing every single
day, you never have to waste energy on deciding whether or not
to do it. Some researchers say that a daily habit is cemented
in as little as 21 days, while others argue that it takes
around 66 days for you to really settle into it. Either way,
there's a point at which it becomes a natural part of your
day, when missing out means leaving a noticeable void.*

If, however, you feel overwhelmed and you freeze at the thought of committing to a ritual every single morning, that's fine, too – no one else is counting. If those daily few minutes feel pointless to you and what you really thrive on can only be done a few times a week, then be honest about that, and pat yourself on the back for dedicating those mornings to doing what makes you feel good. There's nothing noble about high standards that stop you before you even get started.

SACRIFICE AND SELF-KINDNESS
Some say that the rewards of ritual don't come without sacrifice. In a modern world, and in the context of self-care, that might just point to the necessity of being willing to let go – of former habits, former subconscious patterns, even a former self. What it doesn't mean is that it must hurt; sacrifice doesn't have to be painful.

In particular, bearing the following three things in mind will provide you with a solid, unfaltering foundation as you continue on your path of discovery of what a ritual of self-care really looks like for you.

Train yourself to recognize self-criticism: The minute you smell it, take a deep breath and remember why you're doing this; connect with that goal or that feeling.

Shake off the self-censure: When you miss a day or the distractions are too persistent, remind yourself that the idea that achievement is the flip side of the same coin as punishment, that a little bit of pain is probably a good thing, comes from a disordered culture that relies on your sense of inadequacy for its survival. It's not what wellness and self-love are about.

Remember that you're only human: Find the joy in starting each day with an act of kindness toward yourself, but also allow yourself a break when you need it. There's strength in picking yourself up after you fall – with compassion and love, without judgment. Your morning ritual can help you do that. Tomorrow, and the day after tomorrow, and the day after that. Up, and up again, a little stronger every day.

"Our greatest glory is
not in never falling,
but in rising every
time we fall."
— CONFUCIUS

The importance of honesty

Whatever you do, don't set goals because your
parents would have wanted them for you, or
visualize success through the eyes of your
peers. The whole point of a morning ritual is
that it's just for you, so try to find what
makes you feel good and make sure that you
listen to yourself. Don't worry if you make a
mess - you can always start afresh tomorrow.

REFERENCES

Introduction

p11 similar effect on the brain to taking antidepressants A Korb, *The Upward Spiral: Using Neuroscience to Reverse the Course of Depression, One Small Change at a Time* (Oakland, CA: New Harbinger, 2015).

p16 around 11pm when melatonin (a hormone that regulates sleep) peaks H J Lynch et al., "Daily Rhythm in Human Urinary Melatonin", retrieved from https://www.ncbi. nlm.nih.gov/pubmed/1167425; and A F Sigurdsson, "Melatonin – 15 Questions and Answers About Melatonin and Sleep", retrieved from https://www.docsopinion. com/2018/04/02/melatonin-sleep-melatonin-supplements/.

p16 all sorts of negative effects California Department of Public Health, "How to Reduce Exposure to Radiofrequency Energy from Cell Phones", retrieved from https://www.cdph. ca.gov/Programs/CCDPHP/DEODC/EHIB/CDPH%20 Document%20Library/Cell-Phone-Guidance.pdf.

Commit

p25 a podcast that I listened to recently S Parkman and S Ohlanders, "Sommar i P1", retrieved from https:// sverigesradio.se/sida/avsnitt/1077321?programid=2071.

p25 as some scholars have argued C Bell, *Ritual Theory, Ritual Practice* (Oxford: Oxford University Press, 2009).

Breathe

p34 Mindful breathing has been proved to help N Weinstein et al., "A Multi-method Examination of the Effects of Mindfulness on Stress Attribution, Coping, and Emotional Well-being", retrieved from https://greatergood. berkeley.edu/images/uploads/Weinstein-MindfulnessStress. pdf; and M C Melnychuk et al., "Coupling of Respiration and Attention via the Locus Coeruleus: Effects of Meditation and Pranayama", retrieved from https://onlinelibrary.wiley.com/ doi/10.1111/psyp.13091.

p34 Researchers have also found links E Tharion et al., "Influence of Deep Breathing Exercise on Spontaneous Respiratory Rate and Heart Rate Variability: A Randomised Controlled Trial in Healthy Subjects", retrieved from https:// www.ncbi.nlm.nih.gov/pubmed/23029969; and E Grossman et al., "Breathing-control Lowers Blood Pressure", retrieved from https://www.ncbi.nlm.nih.gov/pubmed/11319675.

p37 The vagus nerve B G Bullock, "Tapping into the Power of the Vagus Nerve – How Your Breath Can Change Your Relationships", retrieved from https://www.yogauonline. com/yoga-for-stress-relief/tapping-power-vagus-nerve-how-your-breath-can-change-your-relationships; and C Bergland, "Diaphragmatic Breathing Exercises and Your Vagus Nerve", retrieved from https://www.psychologytoday.com/us/blog/ the-athletes-way/201705/diaphragmatic-breathing-exercises-and-your-vagus-nerve.

p41 many benefits of meditation M Goyal et al., "Meditation Programs for Psychological Stress and Well-Being", *Comparative Effectiveness Review*, No. 124, retrieved from www.effectivehealthcare.ahrq.gov/reports/final.

cfm; B K Hölzel et al., "Mindfulness Practice Leads to Increases in Regional Brain Gray Matter Density", retrieved from https://www.sciencedirect.com/science/article/pii/ S092549271000288X; and "Meditation Offers Significant Heart Benefits", *Harvard Health Letter*, retrieved from https://www. health.harvard.edu/heart-health/meditation-offers-significant-heart-benefits.

p41 people who meditate regularly need less sleep P Kaul et al., "Meditation Acutely Improves Psychomotor Vigilance and May Decrease Sleep Need", retrieved from https://www.ncbi.nlm.nih.gov/pmc/articles/PMC2919439/.

p41 neuroscientific explanation E Mohandas, "Neurobiology of Spirituality", retrieved from https://www. ncbi.nlm.nih.gov/pmc/articles/PMC3190564/; and T Esch, "The Neurobiology of Meditation and Mindfulness", retrieved from https://www.researchgate.net/publication/259263009_ The_Neurobiology_of_Meditation_and_Mindfulness.

Awaken

p64 beneficial knock-on effects Mental Health Foundation, "Let's Get Physical: The Impact of Physical Activity on Wellbeing", retrieved from https://www. mentalhealth.org.uk/sites/default/files/lets-get-physical-report.pdf.

p64 Just 20 minutes is enough to change L Laczo, "How Your Body Changes Once You Start Exercising", retrieved from https://shapescale.com/blog/fitness/exercising/ how-your-body-changes-once-you-start-exercising/.

p67 morning workouts are likely to contribute to a good night's sleep C Price Persson, "Exercise in the morning and sleep better at night", retrieved from http://sciencenordic. com/exercise-morning-and-sleep-better-night.

p67 according to a Bristol University study J C Coulson et al., "Exercising at Work and Self-reported Work Performance", Bristol, UK: University of Bristol, 2008.

p78 helps relieve symptoms of chronic stress J S Feinstein et al., "Examining the Short-term Anxiolytic and Antidepressant Effect of Floatation-REST", retrieved from https://www.ncbi.nlm.nih.gov/pmc/articles/PMC5796691/; and A Kjellgren and J Westman, "Beneficial Effects of Treatment with Sensory Isolation in Flotation-tank as a Preventive Health-care Intervention – a Randomized Controlled Pilot Trial", retrieved from https://www.ncbi.nlm.nih.gov/pmc/ articles/PMC4219027/.

Focus

p91 thinking about the things in life that you are grateful for J Wong and J Brown, "How Gratitude Changes You and Your Brain", retrieved from https://greatergood. berkeley.edu/article/item/how_gratitude_changes_you_and_ your_brain; A Korb, *Upward Spiral: Using Neuroscience to Reverse the Course of Depression, One Small Change at a Time* (Oakland, CA: New Harbinger, 2015); and G A Fox et al., "Neural Correlates of Gratitude", retrieved from https://www. ncbi.nlm.nih.gov/pmc/articles/PMC4588123/.

Nourish

p110 reduces your heart rate and increases blood flow to the brain B M Popkin, "Water, Hydration and Health", retrieved from https://www.ncbi.nlm.nih.gov/pmc/articles/ PMC2908954/.

p113   **psychological consequences of food restriction** J Polivy, "Psychological Consequences of Food Restriction", retrieved from https://www.ncbi.nlm.nih.gov/pubmed/8655907.

p121   **The benefits include optimized metabolism** C Zauner et al., "Resting Energy Expenditure in Short-term Starvation is Increased as a Result of an Increase in Norepinephrine", retrieved from https://www.ncbi.nlm.nih.gov/pubmed/10837292.

p122   **our breakfast choices influence our sleep** M-P St-Onge et al., "Fiber and Saturated Fat are Associated with Sleep Arousals and Slow Wave Sleep", retrieved from https://www.ncbi.nlm.nih.gov/pmc/articles/PMC4702189/.

p122   **Studies have shown that, if we rush a meal** American Heart Association, "Gobbling your Food may Harm your Waistline and Heart", retrieved from https://www.eurekalert.org/pub_releases/2017-11/aha-gyf110317.php; and Institute for the Psychology of Eating, "4 Ways that Stress Impacts Digestion", retrieved from http://psychologyofeating.com/4-ways-stress-impacts-digestion/.

Cleanse

p135   **ice-cold showers are said to strengthen** A Mooventhan and L Nivethitha, "Scientific Evidence-Based Effects of Hydrotherapy on Various Systems of the Body", retrieved from https://www.ncbi.nlm.nih.gov/pmc/articles/PMC4049052/.

p135   **possibly boost productivity** G A Buijze et al., "The Effect of Cold Showering on Health and Work: A Randomized Controlled Trial", retrieved from https://journals.plos.org/plosone/article?id=10.1371/journal.pone.0161749.

Connect

p147   **a proven way to boost happiness** J Zorthian, "More Evidence that Owning a Dog is Really Good for You", retrieved from http://time.com/collection/guide-to-happiness/4870796/dog-owners-benefits/.

p148   **Look to science** J Lee et al., "Restorative Effects of Viewing Real Forest Landscapes, Based on a Comparison with Urban Landscapes", retrieved from https://www.tandfonline.com/doi/abs/10.1080/02827580902903341?scroll=top&needAccess=true&journalCode=sfor20; Y Tsunetsugu et al., "Physiological Effects of Shinrin-yoku [taking in the atmosphere of the forest] in an Old-growth Broadleaf Forest in Yamagata Prefecture, Japan", retrieved from https://www.ncbi.nlm.nih.gov/pubmed/17435356/; and J E Stellar, "Positive Affect and Markers of Inflammation: Discrete Positive Emotions Predict Lower Levels of Inflammatory Cytokines", retrieved from https://www.ncbi.nlm.nih.gov/pubmed/25603133.

p148   **A good dose of vitamin D** "A Prescription for Better Health: Go Alfresco, *Harvard Health Letter*, retrieved from https://www.health.harvard.edu/newsletter_article/a-prescription-for-better-health-go-alfresco; R C Strange et al., "Metabolic Syndrome: A Review of the Role of Vitamin D in Mediating Susceptibility and Outcome", retrieved from https://www.ncbi.nlm.nih.gov/pmc/articles/PMC4499524/; and R Nair and A Maseeh, "Vitamin D: The "Sunshine" Vitamin, retrieved from https://www.ncbi.nlm.nih.gov/pmc/articles/PMC3356951/.

p148   **daylight can boost your melatonin levels** J Douillard, "How Sun Exposure Affects Sleep and Melatonin Production", retrieved from https://lifespa.com/how-sun-exposure-affects-sleep-and-melatonin-production/.

p148   **living near green areas** T Takano et al., "Urban Residential Environments and Senior Citizens' Longevity in Megacity Areas: The Importance of Walkable Green Spaces", retrieved from https://jech.bmj.com/content/56/12/913.

p148   **getting closer to nature** I Alcock et al., "Longitudinal Effects on Mental Health of Moving to Greener and Less Green Urban Areas", retrieved from https://pubs.acs.org/doi/abs/10.1021/es403688w

p148   **the very mechanism** Q Li, et al., "Phytoncides [wood essential oils] Induce Human Natural Killer Cell Activity", retrieved from https://www.ncbi.nlm.nih.gov/pubmed/16873099

p148   **an increased sense of awe** M N Shiota and D Keltner, "The Nature of Awe: Elicitors, Appraisals, and Effects on Self-concept", retrieved from https://greatergood.berkeley.edu/dacherkeltner/docs/shiota.2007.pdf.

p151   **Outdoor exercise boosts your mood and self-esteem** J Barton and J N Pretty, "What is the Best Dose of Nature and Green Exercise for Improving Mental Health? A Multi-study Analysis", retrieved from https://pubs.acs.org/doi/abs/10.1021/es903183r.

p154   **One study from Kansas State University** S-H Park and R H Mattson, "Effects of Flowering and Foliage Plants in Hospital Rooms on Patients Recovering from Abdominal Surgery", retrieved from http://horttech.ashspublications.org/content/18/4/563.full.pdf+html.

p154   **looking at a video of nature scenes** D K Brown et al., "Viewing Nature Scenes Positively Affects Recovery of Autonomic Function Following Acute-Mental Stress", retrieved from https://www.ncbi.nlm.nih.gov/pmc/articles/PMC3699874/.

Trust

p181   **the 3 or 4 hours immediately after 11pm are crucial** S Scutti, "7 Health Consequences of Going to Bed Past Midnight", retrieved from https://www.medicaldaily.com/7-health-consequences-going-bed-past-midnight-247247.

p181   **there are apps to help you** D Nield, "9 Alarm Apps that Will Actually Wake You Up", retrieved from https://www.popsci.com/alarm-apps-wake-up#page-6.

p182   **books have been written on the subject** J Morgenstern, *Never Check Email in the Morning* (New York: Touchstone, 2005).

p182   **productivity experts have identified another problem with it** T Ferriss, *The 4-Hour Work Week* (New York: Crown Publishing Group, 2007).

p186   **Some researchers say that a daily habit is cemented** J Clear, "How Long Does It Actually Take to Form a New Habit? (Backed by Science)", retrieved from https://jamesclear.com/new-habit.

INDEX

PICTURE CREDITS

Alamy Stock Photo Igor Stevanovic 176; Jean-Paul Chassenet 139; Voisin/Phanie 36. **Getty Images** Cultura RM Exclusive/Hugh Whitaker 54; Jochen Schlenker/Robert Harding 24; Malorny 97; Moodboard 46. **iStock** AleksandarNakic 79; alle12 113; ariwasabi 143; Arthur Hidden 175; bigacis 129; bildfokus 23; CasarsaGuru 70; chickaz 146-147; danilovi 186-187; DCC8 98; demaerre 90; deniskomarov 102; Dhoxax 9; dima_sidelnikov 56; dusanpetkovic 61; Eva Katalin Kondoros 125; fizkes 27, 39; flyparade 18; friendwithlove 45; gilaxia 130; gollykim 150; ipopba 58-59; iprogressman 88; itman__47 179; izhairguns 109; Julia_Sudnitskaya 92; Justinreznick 87; laflor 162; Liderina 171; Lifemoment 10; LittleBee80 43; Liubov_Chuiko 120; microgen 49; NadyGinzburg 119; Nastasic 69; Nicola Katie 153; oatawa 80; olindana 141; PeopleImages 17, 35, 83, 101; Peopleimages 105, 116, 183; pixdeluxe 185; SasinParaksa 65; seb_ra 111; SilviaJansen 115; SolStock 161; svetikd 40; Warchi 30. **Jeltje Fotografie**, styling: Cleo Scheulderman 29. **Octopus Publishing Group** Polly Wreford 164; Russell Sadur 134; Ruth Jenkinson 137. **Shutterstock** Suti Stock Photo 66. **Unsplash** Annie Spratt 13; Brittany Neale 155; Casey Horner 157; Darius-Bashar 14; Fachy Marin 169; Naassom Azevedo 149; Sarah Donweller 180; Sven 123.

ACKNOWLEDGMENTS

Writing this book has been a journey for me in more ways than one, and there are a number of people without whom it would never have been written, or completed.

Thank you to Jane Graham-Maw for the clarity and honesty every writer needs from her agent.

To Leanne Bryan, Polly Poulter and Juliette Norsworthy at Octopus for their unending positive energy, expertise and patience.

To Alison Wormleighton for lending her sharp eye and clear thinking, because I meant it when I said that a good copy editor is worth her weight in gold.

To all the people who shared with me their expertise and morning rituals: Aisling Leonard-Curtin, Aisling Twomey, Eva Beronius, Sara Pettersson, Megan C Hayes, Patrick Drake, Jenny Tschiesche, Joanna Nylund, Sophie Hellyer, Rachel Brathen and Claire Baker. I'm grateful for those conversations, and not only because of this book.

To everyone who thought I was mad for taking on this project when I did, but said nothing and allowed me to do things my way – mad or not.

And, finally, to my partner in all of life's and love's lessons, Gary, for always reminding me of what matters and for, as a daily morning meditator, knowing better than most what good mornings are made of.

Thank you.

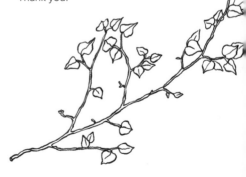